ULTRASOUND GUIDED
'Invasive Prenatal Diagnostic Techniques' Simplified

Raju R Sahetya MD DGO DFP FCPS FICOG
Obstetrician and Gynecologist
Specialist in Infertility, Endoscopy and Prenatal Diagnosis
A Postgraduate from Seth GS Medical College
Mumbai, Maharashtra, India

Forewords

Rustom Phiroze Soonawala MD FRCS FRCOG FICOG
Hema Purandarey MBBS MS FICMH PhD

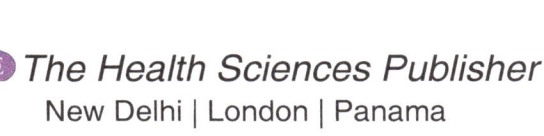

JAYPEE The Health Sciences Publisher
New Delhi | London | Panama

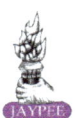 **Jaypee Brothers Medical Publishers (P) Ltd**

Headquarters
Jaypee Brothers Medical Publishers (P) Ltd.
4838/24, Ansari Road, Daryaganj
New Delhi 110 002, India
Phone: +91-11-43574357
Fax: +91-11-43574314
E-mail: jaypee@jaypeebrothers.com

Overseas Offices

JP Medical Ltd.
83, Victoria Street, London
SW1H 0HW (UK)
Phone: +44-20 3170 8910
Fax: +44(0)20 3008 6180
E-mail: info@jpmedpub.com

Jaypee-Highlights Medical Publishers Inc.
City of Knowledge, Bld. 237, Clayton
Panama City, Panama
Phone: +1 507-301-0496
Fax: +1 507-301-0499
E-mail: cservice@jphmedical.com

Jaypee Brothers Medical Publishers (P) Ltd.
17/1-B, Babar Road, Block-B, Shyamoli
Mohammadpur, Dhaka-1207
Bangladesh
Mobile: +08801912003485
E-mail: jaypeedhaka@gmail.com

Jaypee Brothers Medical Publishers (P) Ltd.
Bhotahity, Kathmandu, Nepal
Phone: +977-9741283608
E-mail: kathmandu@jaypeebrothers.com

Website: www.jaypeebrothers.com
Website: www.jaypeedigital.com

© 2018, Jaypee Brothers Medical Publishers

The views and opinions expressed in this book are solely those of the original contributor(s)/author(s) and do not necessarily represent those of editor(s) of the book.

All rights reserved. No part of this publication may be reproduced, stored or transmitted in any form or by any means, electronic, mechanical, photocopying, recording or otherwise, without the prior permission in writing of the publishers.

All brand names and product names used in this book are trade names, service marks, trademarks or registered trademarks of their respective owners. The publisher is not associated with any product or vendor mentioned in this book.

Medical knowledge and practice change constantly. This book is designed to provide accurate, authoritative information about the subject matter in question. However, readers are advised to check the most current information available on procedures included and check information from the manufacturer of each product to be administered, to verify the recommended dose, formula, method and duration of administration, adverse effects and contraindications. It is the responsibility of the practitioner to take all appropriate safety precautions. Neither the publisher nor the author(s)/editor(s) assume any liability for any injury and/or damage to persons or property arising from or related to use of material in this book.

This book is sold on the understanding that the publisher is not engaged in providing professional medical services. If such advice or services are required, the services of a competent medical professional should be sought.

Every effort has been made where necessary to contact holders of copyright to obtain permission to reproduce copyright material. If any have been inadvertently overlooked, the publisher will be pleased to make the necessary arrangements at the first opportunity. The **CD/DVD-ROM** (if any) provided in the sealed envelope with this book is complimentary and free of cost. **Not meant for sale.**

Inquiries for bulk sales may be solicited at: jaypee@jaypeebrothers.com

Ultrasound Guided 'Invasive Prenatal Diagnostic Techniques' Simplified

First Edition: **2018**

ISBN: 978-93-5270-233-6

Printed at:

DISCLAIMER

Medicine is an ever changing science. As new research and clinical experience broaden our knowledge, changes in treatment and drug therapy are required. The author of this book has checked with sources believed to be reliable in their efforts to provide information, that is complete and generally in accord with the standards accepted at the time of publication. However, in view of the possibility of human error or changes in medical sciences, neither the author or the publishers nor any other party who have been involved in the preparation or publication of this work warrants that the information contained herein is in every respect accurate or complete, and he disclaims all responsibilities for any errors or omissions or commissions or duplications or for the results obtained from the use of information contained in this
Ultrasound Guided
'Invasive Prenatal Diagnostic Techniques' Simplified

Raju R Sahetya
MD DGO DFP FCPS FICOG

Dedication

*All those Clinicians and Scientists in Fetal Medicine
who have brought the Technology of Prenatal Diagnosis
as it is today*

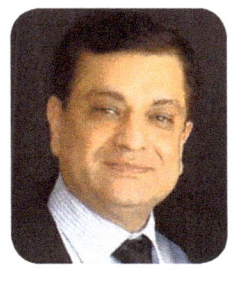

Having have had opportunities to conduct
several 'Workshops'
and 'Hands on Training' in
'Ultrasound Guided — Prenatal Diagnostic Techniques'
I now have a dream to teach these procedures to my practicing colleagues.
The only way I could reach one and all, I thought, was by putting all my experiences in this book
Ultrasound Guided
'Invasive Prenatal Diagnostic Techniques'
Simplified
The emphasis in this book, however is not on theory, but on practical techniques,
and it is anticipated that by following the methods described here,
you too will be able to practice
'Interventional Prenatal Diagnostic Techniques'

Wishing you all the very best

Raju R Sahetya
MD DGO DFP FCPS FICOG

FOREWORD

At present time, preventive medicine is the right approach for good healthcare programmes. This practice in obstetrics has come a long way ever since genetics and ultrasound were introduced in the 1960. The success of cell-free DNA technology, with its high sensitivity and specificity for the detection of trisomy 21, has raised important issues relating to the future conduct of invasive prenatal testing. There is an urgent need to 'future-proof' the safe provision of amniocentesis and chorionic villous sampling (CVS).

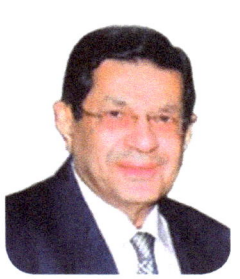

Competency-based assessment and the use of simulation models to reduce the learning curve should be considered as adjuncts to a fixed level of procedural experience. The importance of experienced supervisors in maintaining a safe and effective training environment should be recognized.

I have known Dr Raju R Sahetya now for almost four decades. He is dedicated and committed to learn the newer techniques in practice. I have seen in him, the desire to teach and train all those who attend his 'Hands on Training Workshops' in Ultrasound Guided 'Invasive Prenatal Diagnostic Techniques'.

In his ambition to teach, Dr Raju has reached greater heights by writing this book. He has put in words, the essence of his more than 30 years of experience. He has indeed simplified the invasive techniques for prenatal diagnosis. I am sure the reader will understand and learn the techniques in the right way.

I compliment Dr Raju for a comprehensive and excellent hand book on *Ultrasound Guided 'Invasive Prenatal Diagnostic Techniques' Simplified*

Rustom Phiroze Soonawala
MD FRCS FRCOG FICOG

FOREWORD

The small size of this book has a big scope considering the fact that importance of fetal tissue sampling is the key to various prenatal diagnostic tests even in Genetics and Genomics era.

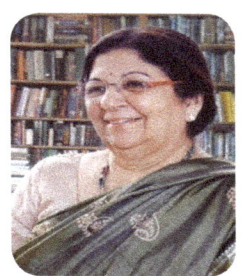

Though every effort is made to offer a pregnant woman, the noninvasive procedure to know the genetic status of her unborn child, the fetal DNA available in maternal blood has yet the limitation of offered tests of aneuploidy screening and certain microdeletions.

The skill required for fetal tissue sampling is described systematically and in details in the chapters 8 to 10. An obstetrician indulging into the practice of diagnosis also requires background and basic knowledge of the laboratory technology available.

Skillful pretest counseling and post-procedure care is being explained in a simplified way in Chapter 4. The ethical issues and the legal aspects are covered in the Chapter 5. Chapters 2 and 3, the paradigm shift in prenatal diagnosis and historical perspectives of diagnostic procedures gives you an insight of evolvement of the techniques required for the fetal tissue sampling.

The author with his personal experience of nearly 3 decades has covered the nuances with the use of low to high resolution technology of fetal tissue sampling. His Chapter 6, covers precise use of ultrasound probes and the principles which any new comer can appreciate and use for safe fetal tissue sampling.

Through this book, the author believes in sharing his skills with the obstetricians interested in fetal medicine, so that more women can avail these facilities without traveling long distances which also add to the risk of fetal wastage.

In india such facilities are not available widely and are rightfully controlled by PCPNDT Act.

I sincerely appreciate efforts of Dr Raju R Sahetya who has explained the right way of doing fetal tissue sampling, which inturn is boon to unborn babies.

Safe mother, safe baby.

Hema Purandarey
MBBS MS FICMH PhD

PREFACE

Antenatal screening identifies those at 'high risk' of fetal consequences, such as aneuploidy, intrauterine infection and fetal anemia, but the diagnosis can only be confirmed or refuted by direct examination of fetal tissue or blood. Until recently, fetal cells could only be obtained by an invasive procedure like amniocentesis, chorionic villous sampling and cordocentesis.

While fetal cells can now be extracted from maternal circulation and analyzed for specific indications, this technique is not widely available and its clinical use remains limited. Invasive technique therefore remains the cornerstone of prenatal diagnosis.

This book focuses on Ultrasound Guided, Invasive Prenatal Diagnostic Techniques. It is essential for established practitioners to have understanding of 'Fetal Medicine' to help answer the question foremost in every prospective patient's mind 'is my baby going to be normal?'.

The Comprehensive Book *Ultrasound Guided 'Invasive Prenatal Diagnostic Techniques' Simplified*

The author is ambitious to train and teach the reader 'Invasive Prenatal Diagnostic Techniques'. In this book, the major indications and variation of Ultrasound guided techniques in 'Fetal Medicine' is covered.

The emphasis of this book, however, is not on theory, but on practical techniques, and it is anticipated that by following the methods described here, one will be able to practice interventional ultrasound guided invasive prenatal diagnostic techniques successfully!

Interventional prenatal diagnostic techniques are not commonly taught at graduate or postgraduate training.

How to reach it well... This is the reason, I decided to write a handbook of techniques covering in one book. I have made every effort to share with every reader all details, description, traps and tricks about the techniques, they should know. I hope this book will be a tool to obstetrician and ultrasonologist, who can refer this book for learning and training and before performing these techniques.

The author has had considerable experience in establishing, performing and training in these techniques to fellow practitioners.

I am indebted to the entire fetal medicine teachers and experts, who have shared their knowledge and expertise from time to time to make this book possible.

Raju R Sahetya
MD DGO DFP FCPS FICOG

ACKNOWLEDGMENTS

I salute Dr Rustom Phiroze Soonawala who has been my mentor and sourse of inspiration.

I thank Dr Hema Purandarey for all the guidance, motivation and direction.

My gratitude Dr S Suresh who has shared his indept knowledge in fetal medicine on many occasion.

My homage to all the pioneers in the field of fetal medicine and in particular— Joley Simpson, Charles Rodeck, Golbus, Ronald Wapner, Diana Bianchi, Brambatti, IC Verma. With whom I had the opportunity to meet, interact and refined my knowledge in Fetal Medicine.

I thank Mr Jitendar P Vij and Ms Payal Bharti of Jaypee Brothers Medical Publishers for their kind cooperation and making this book possible.

CONTENTS

1. **Introduction**   1
   - Who should Undergo Invasive Prenatal Testing   *1*
   - Who can Perform the 'Invasive Prenatal Diagnostic Techniques?'   *3*
   - Diagnostic Techniques Available in Pregnancy   *3*
   - What is the Optimal Prenatal Testing Protocol for Down Syndrome?   *4*

2. **Paradigm Shift in Prenatal Diagnosis**   6

3. **Historical Perspective of Invasive Prenatal Diagnosis: Amniocentesis, Chorionic Villous Sampling, Cordocentesis and Embryoscopy**   10
   - Amniocentesis   *10*
   - Chorionic Villous Sampling (Biopsy)   *12*
   - Cordocentesis and Fetal Blood Sampling   *14*
   - Embryoscopy   *15*

4. **Patient Counseling Prior to Interventional Prenatal Diagnostic Procedures**   16
   - Counseling Prior to Invasive Prenatal Diagnostic Procedure   *16*

5. **Ethical and Legal Issues in Prenatal Diagnosis**   18
   - Ethical Issues   *18*
   - Legal Issues   *19*

6. **Principles of Ultrasound Guided Invasive Prenatal Diagnostic Techniques**   20
   - Technical Aspects   *20*
   - The Ultrasound Principles in Invasive Prenatal Diagnostic Procedure   *23*
   - Visualizing the Needle   *25*
   - Challenges Encountered   *25*
   - Ultrasound Beam   *25*
   - In Plane Technique   *28*
   - Out of Plane Technique   *28*
   - In Plane Approach: Needle Beam Alignment   *29*
   - Align Your Mind   *29*

- Estimating Depth of the Target *30*
- The Tricks and Tips for a Successful Procedure *31*

7. Procedural Prerequisites — 33
- Pregnancy Evaluation *33*
- Clinical Evaluation *33*

8. Amniocentesis — 35
- Principle of Ultrasound: In Plane Approach—Needle Beam Alignment *36*
- Multiple Gestations *39*
- Bloody Tap *41*
- Possible Problems in Amniocentesis *41*
- Amniotic Fluid Sample Collection and Transport to the Genetic Lab *42*
- Cytogenetic Analysis *44*
- Safety *44*

9. Chorionic Villous Sampling — 47
- Procedure Related Anatomy *47*
- Sampling Devices *50*
- Transcervical Chorionic Villous Sampling *52*
- Principles of Ultrasound: The Ultrasound Beam *53*
- Difficulties Encountered and How to Overcome *56*
- Transabdominal CVS *60*
- Complications *62*
- Contraindications *63*
- Timing *63*
- Assessment of Villi Quality *63*

10. Cordocentesis — 66
- Technique *66*
- Complications *67*
- Which Procedure at Which Gestation? *68*

11. Embryoscopy — 70

12. Multiple Pregnancy and Prenatal Diagnosis — 72
- Amniocentesis *72*
- Chorionic Villous Sampling *73*

13. Summary and Suggested Reading — 75
- Summary *75*
- Suggested Reading *77*

Index *79*

CHAPTER 1

Introduction

Many clinical and historical factors can lead to the indications for prenatal diagnosis. Regardless of the specific indication, invasive prenatal testing should be performed with detailed genetic counseling before the procedure. Such counseling is needed to obtain critical information from the patient to assess properly the fetal risk; to review personal and family histories that may have an impact on this risk; to describe the risks, benefits, and limitations of the procedure(s) to be offered; and provide empathetic support to women who are considering such testing.

Genetic counseling should be provided in a nondirective fashion, thus providing women with the necessary information (written and verbal) to arrive at prenatal diagnostic decisions but without coercing the woman, either overtly or covertly, into making a particular decision.

Antenatal screening identifies those pregnancies at 'high-risk' of fetal abnormalities, such as aneuploidy, malformation, intrauterine infections, fetal anemia, but the diagnosis can only be confirmed or ruled out by direct examination of fetal tissue or blood.

Until recently, fetal cells could only be obtained by an invasive procedure: Amniocentesis, Chorionic villous sampling or Cordocentesis. While fetal cells can now be extracted from the maternal circulation and analyzed for specific indications, this technique is not widely available and its clinical use remains limited.

This book Ultrasound Guided 'Invasive Prenatal Diagnostic Techniques' Simplified will focus on training the reader in invasive prenatal diagnostic techniques.

WHO SHOULD UNDERGO INVASIVE PRENATAL TESTING

All pregnant women should be made aware that both diagnostic and screening tests are available for detection of aneuploidy in pregnancy. The majority of women will choose to have screening tests, as this carries no innate risk to her and the pregnancy. She will not wish to discuss diagnostic testing.

For some, the consequences of having a child affected by aneuploidy are of such enormity, that no screening test will give sufficient reassurance. If such concerns are expressed, the mother must have ample opportunity to discuss the full range of diagnostic tests that are available. It is for the women to decide which risk is most acceptable.

The women at increased risk of aneuploidy in pregnancy must be made aware of the risks they are at, and all about the invasive diagnostic techniques. They can then balance the risk of a problem in the pregnancy against the risk of a procedure and make an informed decision on whether or not to proceed with invasive diagnostic technique.

Women who deserve to undergo invasive prenatal diagnostic techniques are those:
1. Women who are at screen 'high-risk'
2. Women or their families with 'specific chromosome abnormality'
3. Ultrasound 'defect in fetus identified'.

Women Who are at Screen 'High-Risk'

A proportion of pregnancies screened for aneuploidy will be classed as 'high-risk'. These need ample opportunity to discuss their individual risk calculation and the diagnostic tests appropriate for their gestational age to rule out of confirm the aneuploidy.

Women or their Families with 'Specific Chromosome Abnormality'

Women or their partners, who carry a balanced chromosome inversion or translocation and are themselves unaffected, are at increased risk of chromosomal abnormities in pregnancy. The fetal medicine team should assess these couples to ensure that the correct risk is calculated, the possible outcomes are understood and the correct diagnostic test is offered to them.

Ultrasound 'Defect in Fetus Identified'

Structural abnormalities in a fetus, such as duodenal atresia, congenital diaphragmatic hernia, cardiac abnormalities, cystic hygroma, holoprosencephaly (HPE), are strongly associated with specific chromosome abnormalities. The risks of aneuploidy will vary, depending on the abnormality identified.

The entire above mentioned patient, high risk for chromosomal abnormality, should undergo invasive prenatal diagnostic technique to visualize chromosomes and to reach an accurate diagnosis (Figs. 1.1A and B).

WHO CAN PERFORM THE 'INVASIVE PRENATAL DIAGNOSTIC TECHNIQUES?'

In India 'Invasive Prenatal Diagnostic Techniques' can be conducted at a center that is registered under the Pre-Conception and Prenatal Diagnostic Techniques (PCPNDT) Act 1994, as Ultrasound and Genetic Clinic. The person performing the procedures should be a registered medical practitioner and should be trained and experienced operator.

DIAGNOSTIC TECHNIQUES AVAILABLE IN PREGNANCY

Women should be given an outline of all the procedures available, the timing of each test and the pregnancy risks associated with each technique, to make an informed decision about prenatal invasive testing. Ideally, these discussions should be supplemented with explanatory booklets that outline the pertinent points and salient statistics. Informed, written consent should be obtained before any testing is performed.

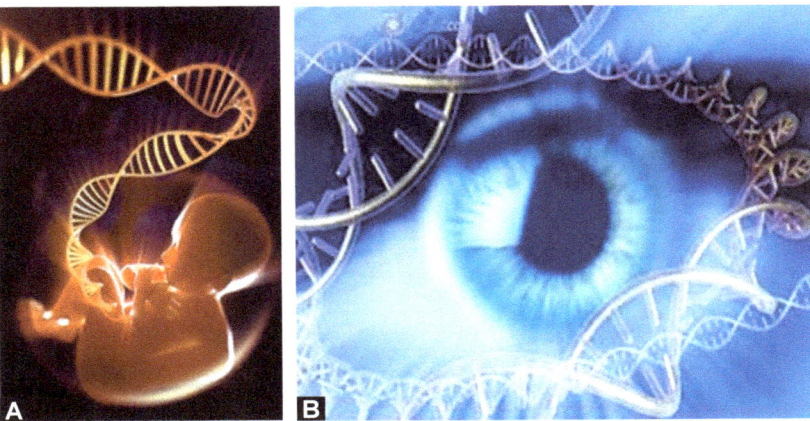

Figs. 1.1A and B: Seeing chromosomes for diagnosis.

WHAT IS THE OPTIMAL PRENATAL TESTING PROTOCOL FOR DOWN SYNDROME?

Here is what the International Society for Prenatal Diagnosis (ISPD) recognizes as the optimal prenatal testing protocol for Down syndrome (Fig. 1.2):

1. Nuchal translucency (NT) test at 11-13 weeks combined with serum markers.

    [ISPD states that 12 weeks is the optimal time for NT testing. ISPD further recognizes that NT is a useful indicator beyond just testing for Down syndrome, e.g. cardiac defects—and says it should be made available separate-and-apart from screening and diagnostic testing for Down syndrome].

2. Offer first trimester (1T) ultrasound (UT) for other soft markers if provider has been validated to perform such testing, e.g. absence of fetal nose bone, tricuspid regurgitation.
3. Contingent test: if Step 1 returns borderline risks, then have Step 2 at a specialist center.
4. Quad test if patient first presents at or after 14 weeks. Though Quad test can be done between 14 and 21 weeks, ISPD recognizes that 15-19 weeks is optimal for also open neural tube screening.

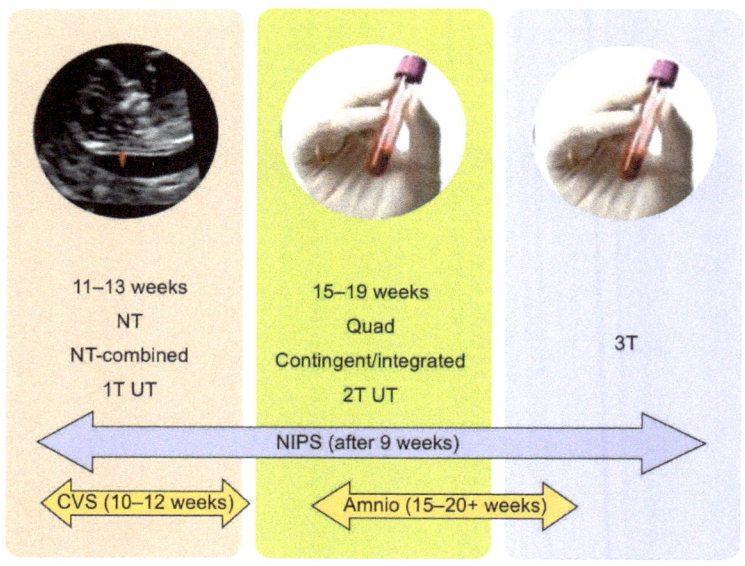

Fig. 1.2: ISPD optimal prenatal testing protocol for Down syndrome.

5. Combine options Step 1 and Step 4 in stepwise or contingent testing provided all screening test data is included in final risk assessment. Only make available integrated screening when chorionic villous sampling (CVS) is not available.

    [Stepwise/contingent is where Step 1 results are reported and then an offer is made to conduct second trimester (2T) quad testing where the results will then be combined; integrated is where Step 1 is performed but results are not reported until 2T test results are returned. Because Integrated has the highest detection rate, American Congress of Obstetricians and Gynaecologists (ACOG) recommends that 'ideally' it should be offered, but it has been criticized on the basis of disrespecting a mother's right to know because it does not report Step 1 results].

6. Contingent 2T UT to modify risks for Steps 1, 4, or 5 results; i.e. like Step 3, if Steps 1, 4, or 5 return borderline risks, have a second trimester 'anomaly scan' performed at 18–23 weeks at a validated center.

    [ISPD further notes that 2T UT, on its own, is 'not a very effective screening test'].

7. Noninvasive Prenatal Screening (NIPS) for high risk women.

    ['High risk' is a result from Steps 1 to 6, or based on maternal age, UT abnormality suggestive of Down syndrome, family history with Down syndrome/aneuploidy, history of previous pregnancy with Down syndrome/aneuploidy].

Step 7 of the ISPD statement is consistent with the previously released guidelines from ACOG and National Society of Genetic Counsellors (NSGC), i.e. NIPS should be offered only to high-risk patients. ISPD makes clear that maternal age alone is insufficient to assess fetal Down syndrome risk other than advanced maternal age being an indicator of high risk for purposes of offering NIPS. Like every other professional guideline, ISPD states that NIPS is not a replacement for amniocentesis or CVS, and only amnio or CVS can provide a definitive diagnosis of Down syndrome.

CHAPTER

Paradigm Shift in Prenatal Diagnosis

The past quarter century has been witness to a series of remarkable advances in the screening of pregnancies for aneuploidy, particularly in the identification of those with Down syndrome.

During the 1970s and early 1980s, advanced maternal age, defined as over 35 years, was the only means by which the general population was assessed as to risk of a fetal chromosomal abnormality.

And of those undergoing invasive prenatal diagnosis only about 2% had fetal karyotype abnormalities, a figure comparable to the 0.5–1% chance of procedure-related fetal loss associated with amniocentesis or chorionic villous sampling (CVS).

In the late 1980s and early 1990s, the introduction of second-trimester maternal serum markers, in the form of 'double', 'triple' and 'quad' marker testing, improved significantly the screening performance for aneuploidy.

The proportion of Down syndrome pregnancies diagnosed more than doubled and a chromosomal abnormality was found in as many as 4% of those designated as 'screen-positive'.

In the late 1990s and early 2000s, aneuploidy screening shifted to the first trimester with the 'combined' test, which uses ultrasound measurement of nuchal translucency thickness (NT) together with maternal serum concentration of placental proteins human chorionic gonadotropin (hCG) (free β, intact or total) and pregnancy-associated plasma protein-A (PAPP-A).

Currently available screening protocols also incorporate additional ultrasound marker, which is Nuchal Translucency (NT).

Consequently, screening performance has improved such that more than nine-tenths of Down syndrome cases can be diagnosed prenatally and the yield from invasive testing has risen to about 6%.

Recently, analysis of cell-free (cff) DNA in maternal blood for noninvasive prenatal testing (NIPT) has been shown to be highly accurate in the detection of common fetal trisomies.

We are in the midst of a paradigm shift in the way that prenatal screening and diagnosis are performed around the world.

This change is occurring in real time at an extremely rapid pace, that is unprecedented in the history of prenatal care. The quest for a less invasive approach to prenatal diagnosis has been the focus of much research over recent decades.

The reason why NIPT represents a paradigm shift is that it changes the algorithm, of screening followed by invasive testing, that has been in practice worldwide for the last 30 years.

Even in the first year of NIPT's integration into clinical care many medical centers are witnessing a significant decline in the number of invasive procedures being performed for aneuploidy.

In addition, every aspect of the current standard of care is being questioned—for example, do we still need to measure maternal serum biomarkers, and what is the place of nuchal translucency measurement?

There is little doubt that tests based on cff DNA provide a readily accessible and generally safer option for prenatal testing that can be offered from 10 until 40 weeks of gestation.

The challenge now is to translate this technology into practice that is accessible to all pregnant women, and in an ethical way that preserves informed parental choice and within the purview of Pre-conception and Prenatal Diagnostic Techniques (PCPNDT) Act 1994, while not increasing overall costs to the heathcare system.

The clinical use of NIPT to screen high-risk patients for fetal aneuploidy is becoming increasingly common. Initial studies have demonstrated high sensitivity and specificity, and there is hope that these tests will result in a reduction of invasive diagnostic procedures as well as their associated risks.

Does that mean 'Invasive Procedures will Disappear?' the answer of course is NO. As a matter of fact the importance of 'invasive prenatal diagnosis' will be on the rise, firstly, one and all who are pregnant will come in the arena of screening and amongst them identifying those at risk above the cut out references, that is 1:100, thereby increasing the number of those deserving prenatal diagnostic tests for confirming the diagnosis will be required, secondly, the reason to do an invasive procedure is perform chromosome microarrays and whole fetal genome studies will be on the rise (Figs. 2.1A and B) the material required for such tests are the amniocytes from large quantity of amniotic fluid and cytotrophoblastic cells culture and mesenchymal cells are harvest, of chorionic tissue obtained by chorionic villous sampling and also of fetal cell derived from fetal blood by cordocentesis.

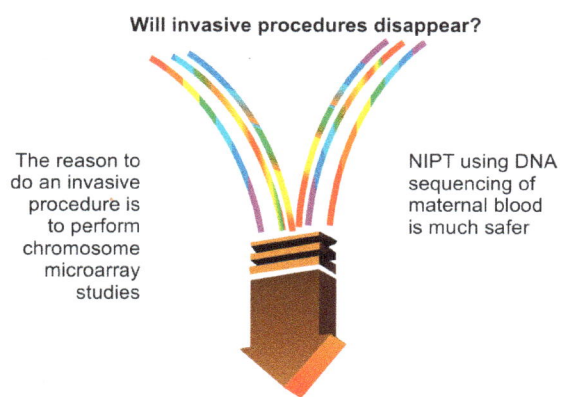

A

B

	Prenatal screening and diagnostic methods			
	Maternal serum screening	NIPT	Chorionic villus sampling (CVS)	Amniocentesis
	Screening tests		Diagnostic tests	
Timing	11–13 weeks and/or 15–22 weeks	≥ 9 weeks	10–12 weeks	15–22 weeks
False positive rate	5%	<1%	<<1%	<<1%
Number of chromosome conditions tested	2–3 conditions T21 T18 and sometimes T13	5+ conditions T21 T18 T13 Monosomy X and Triploidy, SCA Microdeletions*	All chromosomes	All chromosomes
Detailed ultrasound is still recommended for all patients regardless of diagnostic tests				

Figs. 2.1A and B: (A) Future of invasive procedures. (B) Paradigm shift and algorithm for prenatal diagnosis.

Recently, analysis of cell-free (cff) DNA in maternal blood for noninvasive prenatal testing (NIPT) has been shown to be highly accurate in the detection of common fetal trisomies.

We are in the midst of a paradigm shift in the way that prenatal screening and diagnosis are performed around the world.

This change is occurring in real time at an extremely rapid pace, that is unprecedented in the history of prenatal care. The quest for a less invasive approach to prenatal diagnosis has been the focus of much research over recent decades.

The reason why NIPT represents a paradigm shift is that it changes the algorithm, of screening followed by invasive testing, that has been in practice worldwide for the last 30 years.

Even in the first year of NIPT's integration into clinical care many medical centers are witnessing a significant decline in the number of invasive procedures being performed for aneuploidy.

In addition, every aspect of the current standard of care is being questioned—for example, do we still need to measure maternal serum biomarkers, and what is the place of nuchal translucency measurement?

There is little doubt that tests based on cff DNA provide a readily accessible and generally safer option for prenatal testing that can be offered from 10 until 40 weeks of gestation.

The challenge now is to translate this technology into practice that is accessible to all pregnant women, and in an ethical way that preserves informed parental choice and within the purview of Pre-conception and Prenatal Diagnostic Techniques (PCPNDT) Act 1994, while not increasing overall costs to the heathcare system.

The clinical use of NIPT to screen high-risk patients for fetal aneuploidy is becoming increasingly common. Initial studies have demonstrated high sensitivity and specificity, and there is hope that these tests will result in a reduction of invasive diagnostic procedures as well as their associated risks.

Does that mean 'Invasive Procedures will Disappear?' the answer of course is NO. As a matter of fact the importance of 'invasive prenatal diagnosis' will be on the rise, firstly, one and all who are pregnant will come in the arena of screening and amongst them identifying those at risk above the cut out references, that is 1:100, thereby increasing the number of those deserving prenatal diagnostic tests for confirming the diagnosis will be required, secondly, the reason to do an invasive procedure is perform chromosome microarrays and whole fetal genome studies will be on the rise (Figs. 2.1A and B) the material required for such tests are the amniocytes from large quantity of amniotic fluid and cytotrophoblastic cells culture and mesenchymal cells are harvest, of chorionic tissue obtained by chorionic villous sampling and also of fetal cell derived from fetal blood by cordocentesis.

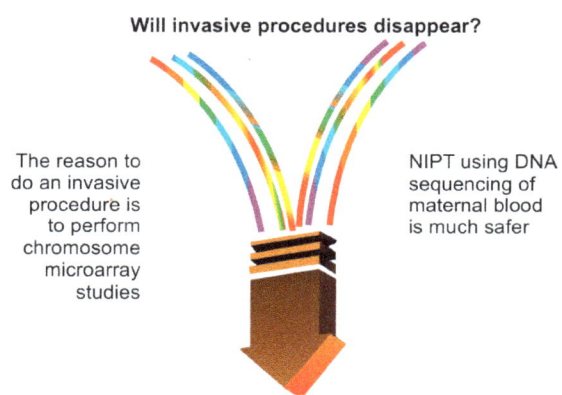

Prenatal screening and diagnostic methods

	Maternal serum screening	NIPT	Chorionic villus sampling (CVS)	Amniocentesis
	Screening tests		Diagnostic tests	
Timing	11–13 weeks and/or 15–22 weeks	≥ 9 weeks	10–12 weeks	15–22 weeks
False positive rate	5%	<1%	<<1%	<<1%
Number of chromosome conditions tested	2–3 conditions T21 T18 and sometimes T13	5+ conditions T21 T18 T13 Monosomy X and Triploidy, SCA Microdeletions*	All chromosomes	All chromosomes

Detailed ultrasound is still recommended for all patients regardless of diagnostic tests

Figs. 2.1A and B: (A) Future of invasive procedures. (B) Paradigm shift and algorithm for prenatal diagnosis.

Therefore Invasive diagnostic procedures are there to be, as in when in late maternal age, with positive family and medical history, when biochemical and or noninvasive prenatal screening (NIPS) tests indicate high risk, and in current scenario for microarray studies and for genomic study of the fetus.

CHAPTER

Historical Perspective of Invasive Prenatal Diagnosis: Amniocentesis, Chorionic Villous Sampling, Cordocentesis and Embryoscopy

AMNIOCENTESIS

Tapping of amniotic fluid had been practised for over a 100 years although many cases had not been recorded. In the literature, transabdominal amniocentesis in the third trimester has been reported by Prochownick, Von Schatz and Lambl in 1877 and Schatz in the 1890s. In 1919 there was a report from Hinkel describing release of amniotic fluid from a patient with polyhydramnios. Menees et al. reported in 1930 removal of amniotic fluid by transabdominal needling. Radiopaque contrast was injected to outline the fetus and placenta. Bevis in 1953 obtained samples of liquor by abdominal paracentesis, at two-weekly intervals, in the management of rhesus isoimmunized patients, and to predict the gravity of the condition.

Liley in Auckland, New Zealand in 1961 published the well-known correlation between the deviation of the spectral absorption curve of liquor amnii resulting from bilirubin, and the severity of rhesus isoimmunization. Since Liley's studies, the practice of amniocentesis had become a standard procedure in obstetric practice.

The first use of amniotic fluid examination in the diagnosis of genetic disease was reported by Fuchs and Riis in 1956 in their seminal article in 'Nature'. They determined fetal sex from cells found in amniotic fluid, basing on the presence or absence of the Barr body. John Edward in England, also discussed for the first time in 1956 the possibility of the 'antenatal detection of hereditary disorders'. The determination of fetal sex led to the prenatal management of patients with Hemophilia A in 1960, and Duchenne muscular dystrophy in 1964.

Steele and Breg very importantly demonstrated in their seminal paper in the Lancet in 1966 that cultured amniotic fluid cells were suitable for karyotyping. Thiede, Creasman and Metcalfe published similar findings later on in the same year. In 1968, Nadler reported on enzyme assays utilizing cultured fetal cells in the amniotic fluid and in the same year reported one of the first diagnoses of Trisomy 21. Their group used cultured cells for a full chromosome analysis. Milunsky and Littlefield discussed the diagnosis of inborn errors of metabolism in 1972. Brock and Sutcliffe in 1972 discovered that excessive amounts of alpha-fetoprotein (AFP) were present in the amniotic fluid of pregnancies with neural tube defects. Other biochemical substances were investigated. Nadler and Gerbie published the important article 'Role of amniocentesis in the intrauterine diagnosis of genetic defects' in the New England Journal of Medicine in 1970. This was the real impetus in genetic amniocentesis and diagnosis, and from then on, genetic laboratories for analysis of amniotic fluid had become prevalent and indications for genetic amniocentesis included the detection of chromosomal abnormalities, X-linked conditions, inborn errors of metabolism, and the neural tube defects.

Gluck et al. in 1971 discovered that fetal lung maturity was found to be related to the surface active phospholipid lecithin. When compared with another phospholipid, sphingomyelin, the lecithin/sphingomyelin ratio was found to be predictive of severe idiopathic respiratory distress syndrome. Ultrasound guidance was started to be employed in amniocentesis with reports from Jens Bang and Allen Northeved from Copenhagen in 1972, where they worked with Hans Hendrik Holm at the Gentofe Hospital, a center which became famous of interventional imaging as early as 1967, and basing on the Vidoson, Hofmann and Hollander in Germany had discussed the importance of placental localization using ultrasound before amniocentesis. Jens Bang and Allen Northeved in Copenhagen described ultrasound-guided amniocentesis in 1972. Prior to the mid-1970s many of the genetic amniocentesis were done 'blind', i.e. the puncture site located merely by external palpation of the uterus in the abdomen. In the mid-1970s to mid-1980s, amniocentesis was performed with the assistance of a static or realtime B-scan. A scan was first performed to locate a feasible pocket of amniotic fluid before a tap, the skin on top of that area was marked and the puncture was done without actually seeing the needle tip going into the fluid pocket. With improving resolution of the realtime scanners, a small number of centers had in the late 1970s started to perform amniocentesis with the simultaneous visualization of the puncture needle tip on the scanner monitor. One such pioneer was the Birnholz group at Harvard who used an early phased array for the purpose. Needle-guide adapters soon became available from ultrasound manufacturers which could be coupled to the linear array or phased array sector probes where the needle passed through a fixed path either parallel or at an angle to the ultrasonic beam. These were cumbersome to use however, particularly in a busy setting. They also had serious problem of keeping the equipment sterile. The adapters may also increase the risk of trauma as it did not allow for the 'desired' and sensitive placement of needles.

Many centers started to do it freehand with an assistant holding onto the transducer probe that was commonly wrapped in a sterile adhesive drape. In 1984, Holzgreve in Basel, Switzerland described a large series of over 3,000 'freehand' amniocentesis with low complication rate. Similar experience was also reported by Platt in Los Angeles, who emphasized on the need for the transducer probe to be manipulated by the same operator which resulted in better hand-eye coordination. In the following year, Romero at Yale formally described the single operator two-hand technique in amniocentesis and the reduction in the number of multiple taps and bloody taps associated with the procedure. Most centers soon adopted the single operator technique, which had become popular because of its convenience and effectiveness. Newer needles were marketed with special external coating and echo-luminance to enhance needle placement. Complication rates were reportedly lower with each successive improvement in technique.

The Benacerraf group reported early amniocentesis (11–14 weeks) in 1988, following some initial reports from Hanson et al. in 1987. In 1990, the Benacerraf group reported an early fetal loss rate of over 2.3%. Several important reviews in the mid-1990s confirmed this high incidence of fetal loss. For this reason, the practice was not met with general acceptance.

CHORIONIC VILLOUS SAMPLING (BIOPSY)

In 1968, Mohr in Scandinavia introduced the concept of antenatal genetic diagnosis using sampled chorionic villi. He performed transcervical biopsy of the chorion under direct endoscopic vision, using a straight 5 mm endoscope. He reported a 96% success rate in obtaining chorionic material but with a high incidence of bleeding, infection and failed culture. The approach was slowly abandoned in the midst of increasing safety from mid-trimester amniocentesis. Kullander and Sandahl in 1973 and Hahnemann in 1974 reported fetal chromosome analysis from transcervical placental biopsy prior to termination in early pregnancies. The first successful prenatal diagnostic use of chorionic villi biopsy was apparently reported in 1975 from the Department of Obstetrics and Gynaecology at the Tietung Hospital in Anshan, China, where fetal sex was diagnosed for the purpose of sex pre-selection. This was reported in the first issue of the (new) Chinese Medical Journal. They performed blind aspirations using a 3 mm metal cannula on a group of 100 patients. When a soft resistance was met, a smaller internal tube was advanced further and placental material obtained by syringe suction. They claimed to have 6 wrong diagnoses out of 99 successful attempts and only 4 prenatal losses. Investigators in the United States were, however unable to duplicate the results and the idea of first trimester antenatal diagnosis was again shelved for some time.

Apparently with the advent of ultrasound and advancement in molecular genetics the desire for an earlier antenatal diagnosis was rekindled. Kazy et al. in 1980, in the USSR reported fetal sexing and enzyme assay on chorion biopsies taken at 6–12 weeks' gestation, using either an endoscopic or ultrasound-guided approach. Biopsy forceps were used instead of cannulas. This was the first report in the literature of using ultrasound guidance during chorion sampling. Niazi et al. in 1981 at the St. Mary's Hospital, London reported improved methods for culturing of fibroblasts from trophoblast villi.

In 1983, Ward in London performed transcervical chorionic sampling under ultrasonic guidance using a 1.5 mm malleable polyethylene catheter and syringe suction. His group reported 67% sampling success rate, including 7 patients for the diagnosis of hemoglobinopathies. The Brambati group in Milan demonstrated in 1983 that with ultrasonic guidance, success rate of obtaining chorionic material rose from 75% to 96%. Brambati used a 1.5 mm polyethylene tube with a soft stainless steel malleable obturator inserted into the 1 mm internal barrel. This design has been the most common design in use today. Other workers like Dumez in Paris used a simple 2 mm biopsy forceps. The Simoni and Brambati group in Milan described in 1983 a technique for direct chromosome and biochemical analysis on first trimester chorionic villi (direct prep), without preliminary culture. Chorionic villi were obtained by aspiration or direct biopsy from the chorion frondosum, at the edge of the placental disc. The inner cytotrophoblastic layer beneath the outer syncytiotrophoblast layer contains actively mitotic cells in freshly sampled villous which could be recovered with their technique. Virtually all analyses could be performed with these fresh whole villous.

In 1984, Smidt-Jensen and Hahnemann in Copenhagen introduced transabdominal fine-needle villous aspiration under ultrasound guidance. With less chance of infective complications and reinsertions the procedure has become more popular than the transcervical counterpart in many prenatal diagnostic centers. Other adjunctive ultrasonic techniques and modifications were reported by the Brambati and Simoni group in Milan and the Golbus group in San Francisco in 1985. The Golbus group reported in 1986 initial experience with 1,000 cases of chorionic villous sampling (CVS) and reported a fetal loss rate of 3.8% and a 1.7% incidence of chromosome mosaicism not found in the fetus. A much lower miscarriage rate of less than 1.5% was subsequently reported by many other centers making the procedure acceptable for routine use.

CORDOCENTESIS AND FETAL BLOOD SAMPLING

After fetoscopy, ultrasound-guided pure fetal blood cordocentesis was pioneered in France in 1983 by Daffos. Pure fetal blood was aspirated in-utero at around 18 weeks from the umbilical vein near the placental insertion of the cord using a 20 gauge needle under ultrasound guidance. Their group reported the first case of Hemophilia A diagnosed in-utero by this method. The procedure was also popularized around the same time in England by the Campbell and Rodeck group at King's College Hospital. The Hobbins group at Yale described their technique in 1985 and called the procedure percutaneous umbilical blood sampling (PUBS). This replaced blood sampling via fetoscopy which the group had pioneered in 1974.

Nicolaides at King's developed the single operator two-hand method and became a leading figure in cordocentesis exploring many important aspects of fetal physiology and pathophysiology. With the advent of color flow mapping, the technique has become even more accessible. In 1988, Nicolini, working with Rodeck at the Queen Charlotte's Maternity Hospital in London, first described fetal blood sampling from the intrahepatic portion of the umbilical vein in the fetus, as an alternative procedure in cases where cord needling was unsuccessful.

EMBRYOSCOPY

In 1990, Cullen, Reece, Whethaam and Hobbins described the new technique of 'Embryoscopy', a transabdominal thin gauge embryofetoscopy procedure in the first trimester. Quintero, Abuhamad, Hobbins and Mahonney reviewed the clinical application of the procedure in 1993 and reported the early prenatal diagnosis of a case of Meckel-Gruber syndrome using this technique.

Patient Counseling Prior to Interventional Prenatal Diagnostic Procedures

This chapter reviews the basic principles of genetic counseling relevant for patients considering undergoing prenatal diagnostic techniques.

Genetic counseling is a communication process which deals with the problem associated with the risk of occurrence of a genetic disorder. An appropriately trained person helps to:
1. Comprehend the medical facts, including the diagnosis and available management.
2. To educate how heredity contributes to the disorder, and the risk of recurrence in relatives.
3. Alternatives for dealing with the risk of recurrence.
4. Action which seems to them appropriate in view of their risk.
5. To make the best possible adjustment to the disorder and to the risk of recurrence.

COUNSELING PRIOR TO INVASIVE PRENATAL DIAGNOSTIC PROCEDURE

Invasive procedures performed during pregnancy differ from procedures performed in any other medical setting since there are two patients potentially at risk, the mother and the fetus. Although the physician's primary obligation is to the mother, he or she must, in pregnancies destined to continue, also do everything possible to safeguard the health of the fetus. There are some circumstances in which there are several alternative procedures available that could potentially accomplish the same reproductive goal with safety.

However, although the goal should be to adhere to a nondirective approach in providing genetic counseling, most experienced counselors are aware that a purely nondirective means may be difficult to achieve. A patient's decision can be significantly influenced in very subtle ways to help her to understand the gravity of situation and to make an informed consent.

Patient Counseling Prior to Interventional Prenatal Diagnostic Procedures

In counseling patients regarding the risks of invasive procedures, it is essential that a discussion of all known risks be accompanied by discussion of what is unknown. Although the emphasis so far in the discussion of counseling patients prior to invasive procedures has focused on risks, both known and unknown, there are many other important components to such counseling. These include a realistic appraisal of possible and likely benefits, accuracy of diagnostic tests to be utilized, and a discussion of alternatives. Also implication in testing verses no testing. The patient must be given the time and opportunity to carefully consider all of the issues related to any such decision before she can truly provide informed consent.

Prior to initiating a procedure during which there may be unanticipated or adverse findings, the physician should consider how this will be addressed with the patient. Although some discussion of the findings may be necessary during the course of the procedure, a detailed discussion is best conducted with the patient at eye level in a face-to-face encounter. In addition to considering the possibility of adverse findings, the physician should also be prepared for the occurrence of complications during invasive procedures and should give thought to how such occurrences will be communicated to the patient.

With regard to the choice between chorionic villous (CVS), and traditional midtrimester amniocentesis, the issue is somewhat more complex since, although the risks associated with CVS are somewhat more than those associated with amniocentesis, the diagnosis is achieved an average of 4–6 weeks earlier in pregnancy and termination in the first trimester is generally easier and has a benefit of privacy than in the second trimester.

Many factors, such as the patient's past pregnancy experiences and the perceived importance of procedure-induced fetal loss or fetal defects, among others, will influence the patient's decision.

CHAPTER

Ethical and Legal Issues in Prenatal Diagnosis

ETHICAL ISSUES

Ethical dilemmas abound prenatal diagnosis and will only grow as the technical capabilities of invasive procedures increase. One of the most significant is when it is ethical for a physician to offer a new invasive technique, with a relatively high or unknown risk, to a patient. The potential for harm is so great in such circumstances, that utmost care should be utilized in arriving at an answer to this question. The burden of responsibility cannot and should not be shifted to the patient by saying that the patient will be told that the risks are unknown.

The very act of offering a procedure to a patient, makes a statement that accepting it is a reasonable choice. Recognizing that some adverse effects may require many years to identify, the burden on the physician to counsel the patient appropriately is very great indeed. The physician must be careful to make a distinction for the patient between what they think the risks may be and what they know.

An ethical dilemma that may arise with increasing frequency in the future relates to the issue of controversial indications for prenatal diagnosis. Another obvious ethical dilemma that arises in any discussion of prenatal diagnosis relates to abortion choices. The physician's own personal views on the abortion issue are irrelevant to the individual patient's decision of what is best for her and for her family. In a society in which abortion is a legal option, the physician is obligated to present it to the patient as an alternative in an objective and nondirective fashion and to support her in whatever decision she makes.

While those patients who choose to terminate an abnormal pregnancy should be provided with maximal support, since their grief and sense of loss is often overwhelming, it is equally important that patients confronted with the diagnosis of a fetal abnormality do not feel compelled by the physician to undergo abortion. Continuation of pregnancy in the face of a fetal abnormality, even a lethal one, must be presented as a valid alternative, although it defeats the purpose of performing invasive prenatal diagnostic procedure.

LEGAL ISSUES

Most malpractice lawsuits involving prenatal diagnosis can be divided into several categories.

The first categories of malpractice include:
1. Failure to obtain, or appropriately respond to, relevant clinical information. This would include failure to obtain an adequate family history or other relevant information leading to failure to identify factors that place the patient at increased risk of a specific birth defect or genetic disorder.
2. Failure to arrive at an accurate diagnosis in a patient who presents with findings that could reasonably lead to a diagnosis.
3. Failure to provide accurate genetic counseling.
4. Failure to offer prenatal diagnosis to patients at increased risk of having a child with a detectable disorder.
5. A closely related but somewhat different allegation would involve the failure to secure fully informed consent prior to a diagnostic procedure.

A second general category of malpractice actions are those alleging negligence in the performance of invasive procedures that result in a complication causing damage to the patient. The patient clearly has a legal right to expect that procedures will be performed using proper equipment by a skilled operator or at least under the supervision of a skilled operator. While it may be difficult in many cases to distinguish a complication that is an inherent risk of a procedure from one resulting from negligence, it is imperative that patients be informed in advance of all known complications that may occur.

The final common category into which malpractice lawsuits related to interventional procedure fall is that involving allegations of error resulting in misdiagnosis or no diagnosis. This encompasses errors occurring within laboratory as well as inappropriate handling of samples before reaching the laboratory. Clearly not all laboratory errors or misdiagnoses are a result of negligence. There are inherent inaccuracies in many of the tests used for prenatal diagnosis. Patients should be clearly informed of the accuracy of individual tests and possible reasons for inaccuracies prior to undergoing any diagnostic procedure.

CHAPTER

Principles of Ultrasound Guided Invasive Prenatal Diagnostic Techniques

Ultrasound-guided invasive procedures initially appear simple but may sometimes prove to be tricky. A two-dimensional image is identified, the target seen and all one simply needs to do is guide the needle percutaneous to the target. However one feels regularly that the procedure was unsuccessful because of inability to visualize the needle all the way along with the tip.

In order to maximize success, the operator must have enough experience to use the correct transducer, the correct instruments and, the proper gain settings, and there must be appropriate coordination between the operator and the sonologist. Above all, the knowledge and principles of ultrasound for guided invasive prenatal diagnostic techniques.

Although amniocentesis is the most commonly used ultrasound-guided procedure in prenatal diagnosis, numerous other procedures have been developed based upon the ability of ultrasound to guide an instrument within the body.

1. Chorionic villous sampling, obtaining ultrasound guided, targeted and avoiding maternal contamination, chorionic villi from the chorionic frondosum, these being live, budding villi, for rapid culture and accurate prenatal diagnosis.
2. Percutaneous umbilical blood sampling (PUBS), also called as cordocentesis, relies on ultrasound guidance of the needle to the umbilical cord, thus allowing for puncture of an umbilical vessel for direct hematological or biochemical analysis of the fetus.
3. Fetoscopy, direct fetal visualization is also guided by ultrasound until the target could be visualized for the purpose of therapy of biopsy.

TECHNICAL ASPECTS

The evolution of amniocentesis techniques over the last quarter of a century provides insight into all invasive procedures.

Principles of Ultrasound Guided Invasive Prenatal Diagnostic Techniques

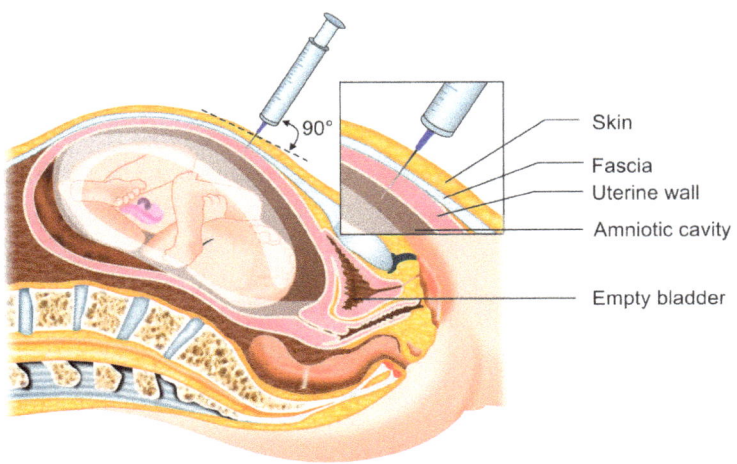

Fig. 6.1: Palpation or Touch technique amniocentesis.

When amniocentesis was originally introduced it was performed in a blind technique. The operator was guided by palpation of the fetus in-utero or the hands-on 'touch technique', where the operator tried to feel the needle crossing the different tissue layers (Fig. 6.1).

With introduction of ultrasound, patients began to present for the procedure with an 'X' on the abdomen where ultrasound determined fluid pocket was discovered. With improvement in skills, equipment and experience, the ultrasound machine and the operator came closer together in time and location. One team was able to identify the fluid pocket and perform the procedure immediately afterwards. Even so, the tendency was to put the transducer down just prior to the procedure.

The final development was that of continuous ultrasound guidance until the needle tip reached the target. This technique allows for instantaneous correction of the needle direction and depth of insertion to take into account the always changing intrauterine enjoinment. To anyone who has participated in this technical evolution it is now practically unthinkable to perform any invasive procedure without continuous ultrasound guidance.

Three variations of the continuous ultrasound-guided procedures exist:
1. In the single-operator technique, a single skilled individual performs the procedure with his/her dominant hand while guided by the transducer held in the other hand. Usually an assistant is made available to withdraw the stylet and aspirate the fetal sample. The 'single-operator technique allows for the closest cooperation between 'scanning' and 'needling' as it is done by the same individual. Unfortunately, this leaves the task of actual aspiration to a frequently uninitiated assistant. This can lead to inadvertent movement or dislodging of the needle at the time of aspiration, thus increasing the hazard of the procedure.
2. The two operator technique is preferred, where a sonologist performs the ultrasound guidance while the operator places the needle. In this way, the operator manipulates the needle with necessary finesse to reach the desired target. This technique is dependent on a close relationship and coordination between the sonologist and the operator. The sonologist and the operator must be able to communicate well and almost to anticipate each other's fine movements.
3. Some operators advocate using a fixed needle guide on the transducer head in order to assure the needle path. This technique however locks the needle and the transducer together, so once the procedure has started the transducer cannot be moved.

There are three free-hand techniques based upon the orientation of the needle and the transducer:
1. The first is a perpendicular offset approach, where the transducer is placed off the sterile sheet field at 90 degrees to the path of the needle. This is only practical with a protuberant or pregnant abdomen. This procedure not found to be very successful, as the distance between the transducer and the target is frequently outside the focal point and length of the transducer.
2. The second technique is frequently referred to as 'parallel' or 'side-on' approach, where the needle is introduced at the midpoint of the side of the transducer. Although this technique usually assures the operator what is below the transducer, it is unlikely to see more than a single point on the needle shaft. The point seen is not necessarily the tip of the needle, but is only the

Principles of Ultrasound Guided Invasive Prenatal Diagnostic Techniques

position where the needle shaft crosses the plane of the ultrasound beam.
3. The third technique an 'end-on' approach to ultrasound beam is the most successful method. With this technique the target is identified and the needle is introduced at the short end of the transducer. The angle of entry can vary and the transducer can be rocked along the abdominal wall. It is important, however, for the operator to be familiar with the focal plane of the transducer.

Before leaving the technical issue of invasive procedures we should address the issue of optimizing machine settings in order to enhance visualization. The gain setting should be adequate enough to visualize the instrument or needle that is being advanced towards the target.

Maintaining sterility in ultrasound-guided procedures is of paramount importance to avoid postprocedure infections.

Another prerequisite for invasive procedures is that the operator should have extensive experience in ultrasound scanning; although it is possible for the operator to be guided by another sonologist, coordination is inevitably better one brain, rather than two.

Invasive procedures can be performed with curvilinear transducers because it combines the advantages of both linear-array and sector systems (the needle is visualized throughout its length and the image of the tip is sharp). Furthermore, the free-hand technique is preferred because it allows freedom for manipulation, if the position of the target is suddenly altered by a uterine contraction or fetal movements.

THE ULTRASOUND PRINCIPLES IN INVASIVE PRENATAL DIAGNOSTIC PROCEDURE

While performing ultrasound guided prenatal diagnosis technique, one has to have complex orientation and coordination of the following (Fig. 6.2):
1. The probe
2. The target
3. The needle

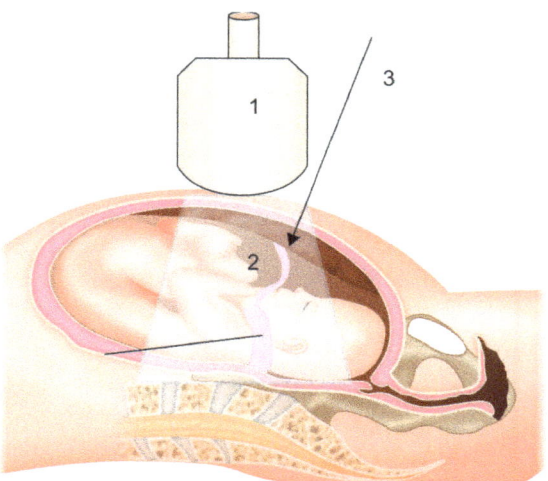

Fig. 6.2: Coordination of the probe, the target and the needle.

The rule is that, during the procedure only one of these three can move, other two remain static.

1. **The probe** moves and after necessary evaluation, orientation of the procedure and localization of the target has to be stabilized and should not move. This is possible if the probe is gently applied to the contact surface and the conducting ultrasound-gel is adequate and not in excess. If pressure is applied with excess gel, not only is it responsible for the pain but also the transducer often glides on the curvature of the abdominal wall due to the globular contour of the pregnant uterus and losses the orientation and localization of the target.
2. **The target** often is localized, and after ascertaining that it is free of the fetal parts, loops of umbilical and all other important structures that may lead to an eventful procedure. Therefore it is very important that the fetus does not move and you have a complication free successful procedure. If the fetus moves and loops of umbilical cord are seen appearing at or on way to the target, one has to re-evaluate and reorient before the procedure.
3. **The needle**, moves after reassuring that the target has been finalized and fetus and all other important structures are out of path and target, once the needle penetrates and proceeds to the target, the probe just cannot be moved as the ultrasound probe

Principles of Ultrasound Guided Invasive Prenatal Diagnostic Techniques

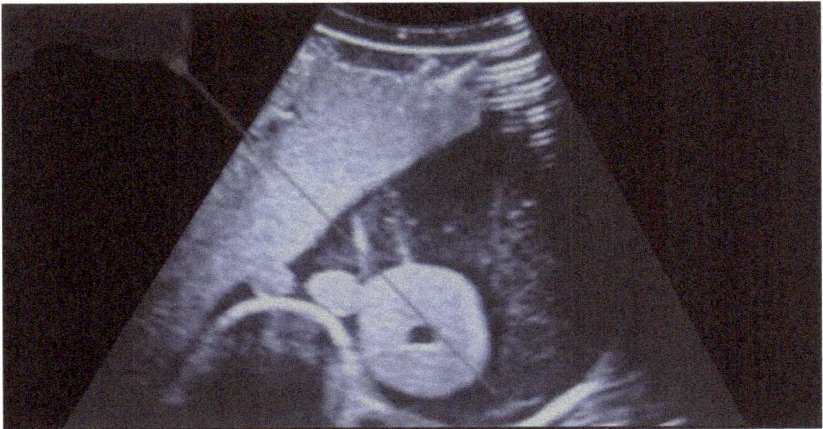

Fig. 6.3: Visualizing the needle all the way.

is guiding the needle to the target, and it is very important that the entire needle, the shaft and more, so the tip of the needle is clearly visualized at all time until the target is reached.

VISUALIZING THE NEEDLE

The needle has to be visualized throughout the procedure, at the entry, towards the target, reaching the target and at the time of exit of the needle (Fig. 6.3). When these steps are followed, it truly defines and means that you have performed an ultrasound guided procedure.

CHALLENGES ENCOUNTERED

The most frequent challenge encountered is the location of the target; the target could be located in the center and superficial, on side, right or left or could be far and posterior (Fig. 6.4). Accordingly the approachability could be anterior, lateral or posterior. The most suitable entry points are anterior and lateral approach (Fig. 6.5). The vital structures coming in the path should be visualized and avoided. The rule therefore is to scan and plan the procedure.

ULTRASOUND BEAM

Understanding the ultrasound beam is of utmost importance. The thickness of the beam is limited to the thickness and stretch of the

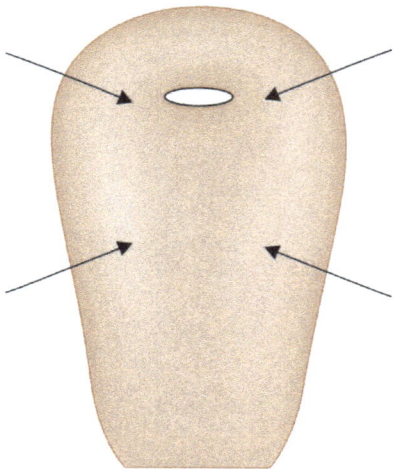

Fig. 6.4: Location of target anterior, lateral or posterior.

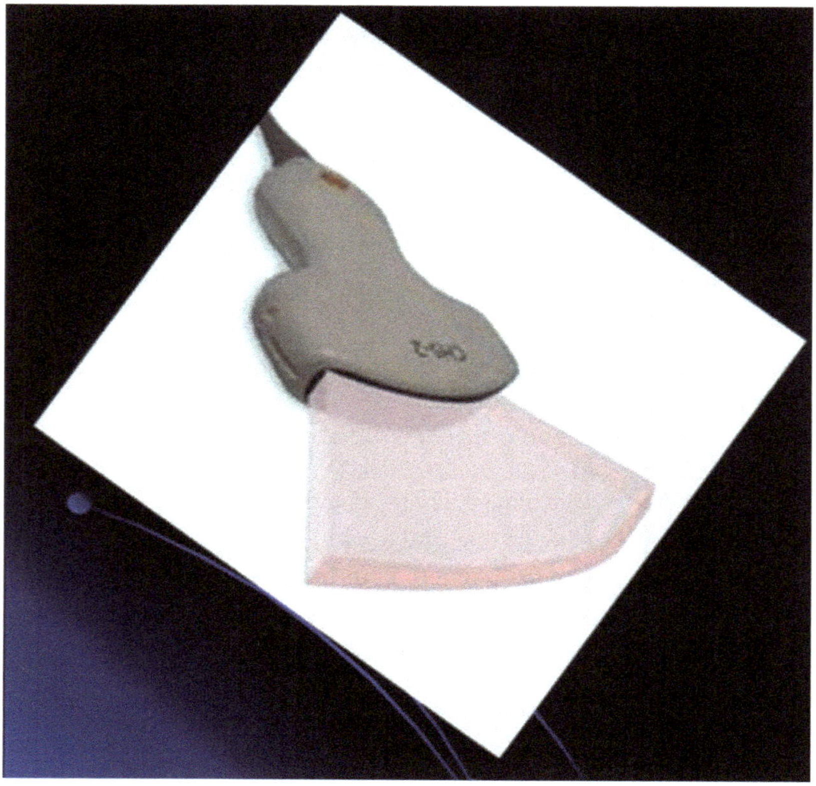

Fig. 6.5: Anterior and lateral approach.

Principles of Ultrasound Guided Invasive Prenatal Diagnostic Techniques

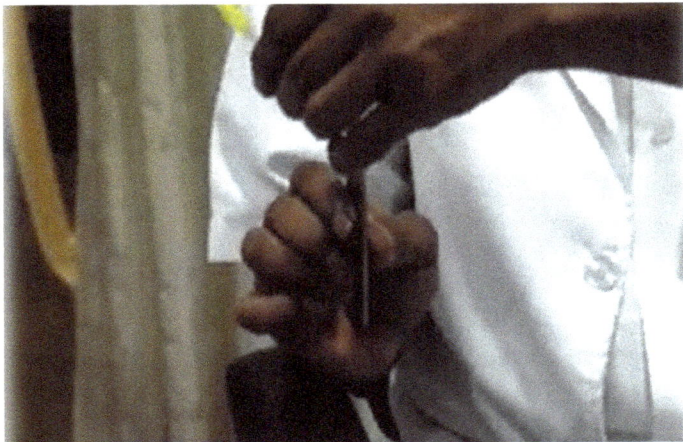

Fig. 6.6: Demonstration of the ultrasound beam.

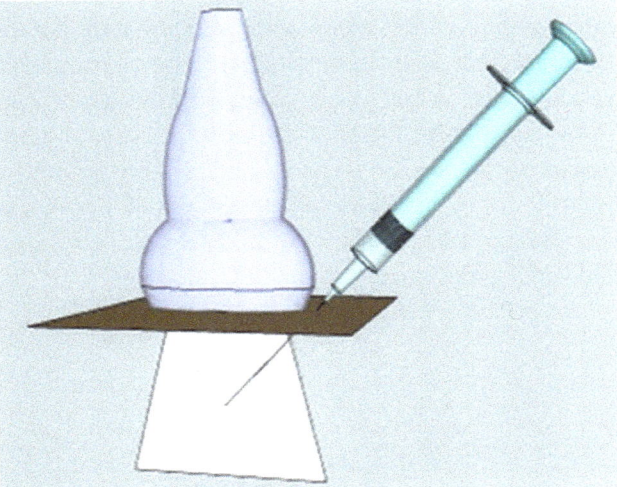

Fig. 6.7: Aligning the ultrasound beam.

rubberized portion of the curved surface of the curvilinear probe forming a segment of visualizing surface (Fig. 6.6). This is comparable to visual restriction by the two eye lids to the ability of the eye to visualize. Only if the needle is placed in this segment, it can be visualized at all time during the procedure by the guiding ultrasound transducer. Therefore it is all about aligning the ultrasound beam and needle (Fig. 6.7).

IN PLANE TECHNIQUE

The transducer is held by the fingers of the nondominant hand and needle is firmly held between the thumb and the index finger of the dominant hand at the entry point at one end of the transducer and within the thickness of the transducer beam. For the needle to be visualized entirely, the needle is directed at 45° to the imaginary line on the center of the flat of the transducer, so that the needle traverses all the way beneath the thickness of the transducer and therefore within the ultrasound beam (Fig. 6.8). This technique enables visualization of the entire needle, the shaft and the tip as the needle is guided while moving towards the target.

OUT OF PLANE TECHNIQUE

In this the point of entry is along the flat surface of the transducer and the long-axis of the needle in a plane perpendicular to the ultrasound beam and the cross-sectional area of the needle is imaged (Fig. 6.9). This technique results in poor visualization of the needle, as the angle of approach being parallel to the transducer therefore may almost be parallel to the ultrasound beam. Only a short segment of the needle is visualized as only a small segment of the needle is imaged. What we may think as tip of the needle may be the shaft of the needle. This may result into complicated and unsuccessful procedure.

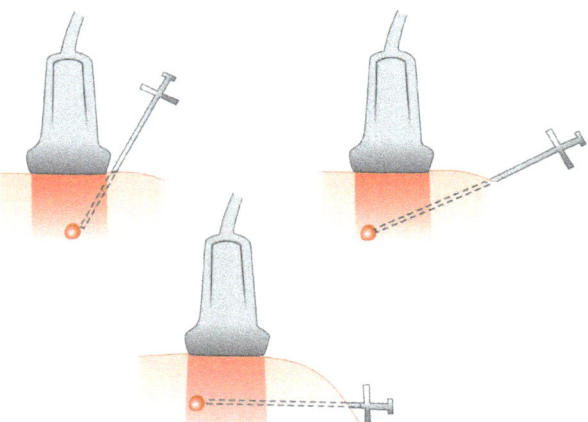

Fig. 6.8: In plane technique.

Principles of Ultrasound Guided Invasive Prenatal Diagnostic Techniques 29

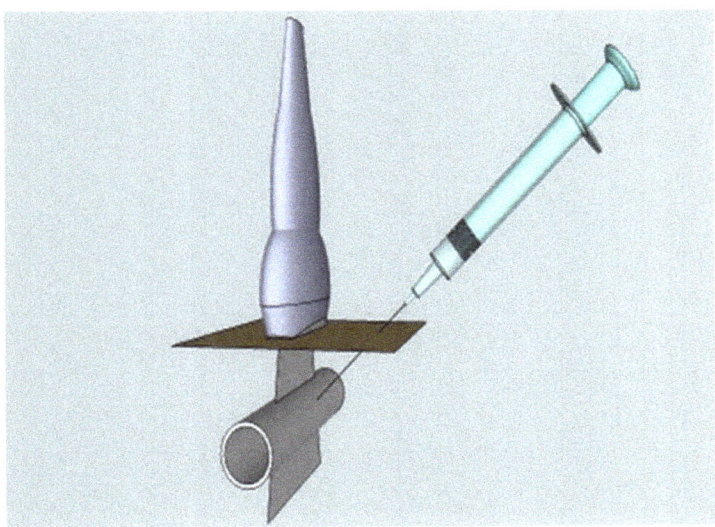

Fig. 6.9: Out of plane technique.

IN PLANE APPROACH: NEEDLE BEAM ALIGNMENT

Needle beam alignment is very important and best achieved when needle is inserted in the same plane as ultrasound beam, this enables needle to be visible as a bright line, needle beam alignment is critical to visualize the entire shaft up to the tip of the needle. Needle should be advanced well-guided and at an angle of 45° or less depending on the location of the target (Fig. 6.10).

During the procedure, if the needle is lost, first stop advancing the needle. Locate needle by angulations of the probe, move probe and identify needle tip, finally move probe and needle together, under vision, back in line to the target (Fig. 6.11). Thereafter fix the transducer and then advance the needle as you see it, deeper you go, tracking and manipulating the needle will be painful, traumatic and difficult, therefore orient and angulated the needle at the entry point. Always remember to maintain the 45° angle while advancing the needle.

ALIGN YOUR MIND

It is all about aligning your mind to all the variables, the probe, the target and the needle. The operator's skill in aligning the probe and the needle is the most important variable influencing the

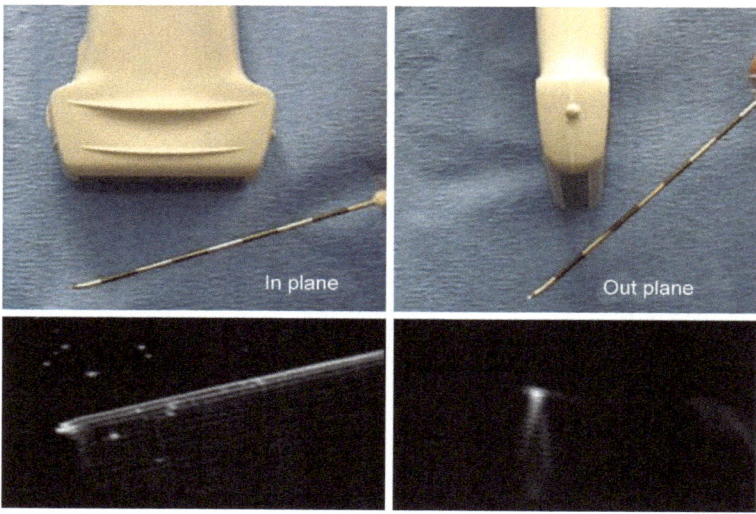

Fig. 6.10: In plane and out of plane images.

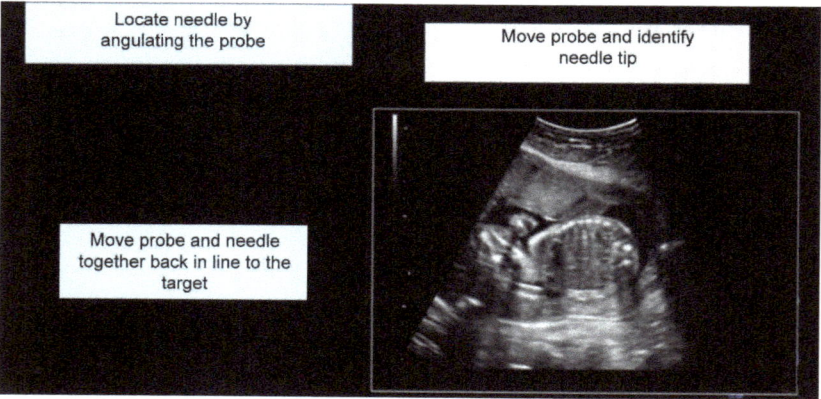

Fig. 6.11: Tips and tricks when needle is lost during procedure.

needle visualization and resulting into an uneventful, atraumatic, uncomplicated technique, resulting into adequate sampling and a successful procedure.

ESTIMATING DEPTH OF THE TARGET

It is very important to estimate the depth, where targeted biopsy like that of the shin of the bone, muscle, etc or in the procedure of Intra uterine transfusion, selective fetal reduction and likewise procedures (Fig. 6.12).

Principles of Ultrasound Guided Invasive Prenatal Diagnostic Techniques

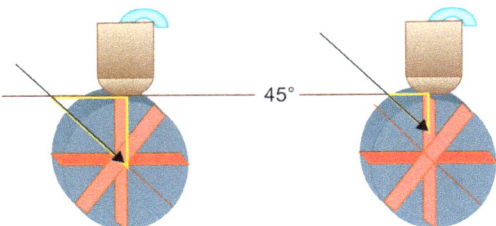

Fig. 6.12: Estimate of depth to reach the target.

After ultrasound evaluation and measurement of the depth of to the target, the point of insertion is estimated, by measuring the same distance as the depth of the target, and away from the imaginary point on the center of the flat and outer surface of the transducer. The angle of insertion has to be maintained at 45° to meet the imaginary vertical line drawn downwards to the target. The distance of the target and to point of insertion on the skin are the same, making an 'An right angle triangle, having right angle at the point of contact with the transducer, having all three sides equal and has two angles each at 45°'.

THE TRICKS AND TIPS FOR A SUCCESSFUL PROCEDURE

There is a general lack of literature or 'Hand Book' on Invasive Techniques for Prenatal Diagnosis, therefore a conventional obstetrician is not exposed to reading, seeing or performing these procedures. There are counted few who have taken an informal training and practice these techniques on regular basis at the specialized center for prenatal diagnosis and genetics. Like any other procedures, skills are acquired through practice and opportunities available for experiences are limited.

Many more can be trained in invasive prenatal diagnostic techniques, if one follows the principle 'see one, do one, teach one. Those who know the art of ultrasound, the diagnosis and ultrasound guided procedure and learn and master the procedures precisely. Although one uses 2D ultrasound machines for the invasive techniques, one has to visualize as if 3D in the mind.

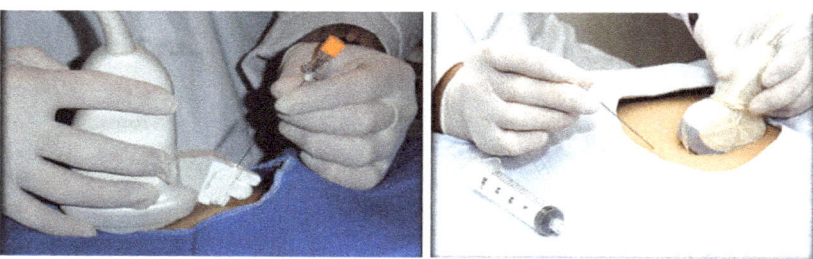

Fig. 6.13: Needle directed at 45° using biopsy guide/free hand technique.

For a successful Invasive diagnostic technique, always scan just before you start the procedure. Identify the target, recognize the intervening structures. Procedure orientation is very important. This helps to decide on the type and length of the needle or shape of the performed, malleable cannula, as in the procedure of transcervical chorionic villous sampling.

The transducer is held in the left hand of a right handed operator, the desired target is identified and the transducer is aligned in such a way that the target is in the center of the screen while the proposed site of entry in the maternal abdomen is visualized at the edge of the screen. Subsequently, the right index finger is placed on the maternal abdomen, about 2–3 cm away from the edge of the transducer, and pressed firmly towards the uterus. Provided the finger and the transducer are within the same plane, the indentation caused is clearly visible, allowing the operator to simulate needle insertion. The needle or instrument is then introduced into the uterus, ensuring that the whole length is visualized continuously. This is best achieved when the needle is directed at 45° from the horizontal plane of the transducer (Fig. 6.13).

CHAPTER 7

Procedural Prerequisites

After relevant counseling and obtaining informed, written consent, pregnancy is evaluated to decide the time, method and route of approach for the invasive prenatal diagnosis test.

PREGNANCY EVALUATION

Genetic Counseling

Indication for referral reviewed, alternate procedure discussed, risks complications and advantages explained, testing versus no testing counseled and thereafter informed written consent obtained.

CLINICAL EVALUATION

A detailed obstetric history is very essential, number of pregnancies, number of living children, importantly number of miscarriages. These details categorize the patient as low or high risk for the invasive procedures.

Genital infection should be checked for and ruled out, if present, more so for the transcervical technique should be treated before the procedure, as they pose high risk of being carried intrauterine during the procedure and make the procedure high risk for pregnancy loss.

Recent bleeding in current pregnancy should be asked for and if so, one has to evaluate the causes for it; the patient may be at risk of spontaneously aborting even without the procedure. Also such pregnancies are at high risk for aneuploidy.

Ultrasound Evaluation

This is of utmost importance, to determine fetal gestational age and viability.

If multiple gestations are detected, viability and age of both are checked for. One has to keep in mind the possibilities of vanishing of one of the twins and the same has to be counseled with the patient.

Chorionic frondosum is identified by visualizing the site of cord insertion. Localizing and mapping the chorionic frondosum is very important as viable, budding villi, easy to obtain and culture in the lab and study for prenatal diagnosis are obtained only.

Subchorionic bleeding/hematoma ruled out. Uterocervical relation is evaluated. Whether the uterus anteverted or anteverted-anteflexed. This will require adequate bladder for correction of anteverion-anteflexion in transcervical chorionic villi sampling. In retroflexed retroverted uterus one should restrict bladder size to minimal requirement as for acoustic window otherwise the mobility would get restricted and maneuvering of the transcervical cannula not only difficult but impossible.

The most important of ultrasound evaluation is the orientation of the entire procedure. One can visualize, orienting for the entire journey of the needle or cannula towards the target for procedure of biopsy.

Ultrasound evaluation helps to decide the route of approach, the length of the needle or cannula and also helps to preform and shape the malleable cannula as for the transcervical procedures (Fig. 7.1).

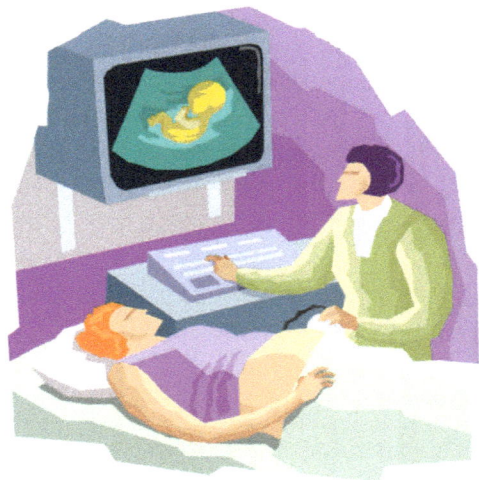

Fig. 7.1: Ultrasound evaluation preprocedure.

CHAPTER 8

Amniocentesis

Midtrimester amniocentesis, the aspiration of amniotic fluid, has traditionally been performed between 15 and 18 weeks of gestation. At this stage of gestation, the volume of amniotic fluid is about 200 mL. The ratio of viable to nonviable cells in the amniotic fluid is relatively high, thus allowing timely culture and diagnosis of fetal cytogenetic abnormalities and providing women the option of pregnancy termination should an abnormality be determined.

Amniocentesis is routinely an outpatient facility and an ultrasound-guided procedure. Having confirmed fetal viability, an accessible pool of amniotic fluid should be determined (Fig. 8.1). Ideally passage through the placenta should be avoided but, if this is not achievable, a transplacental approach may be employed. If a transplacental tap is necessary, the thinnest portion of placenta, avoiding the cord insertion point, should be selected.

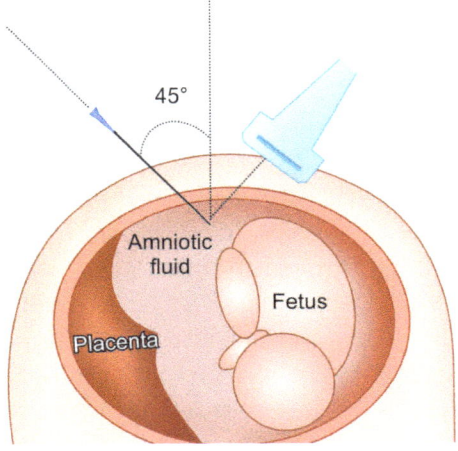

Fig. 8.1: Locating amniotic pocket.

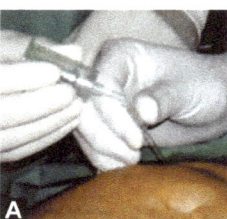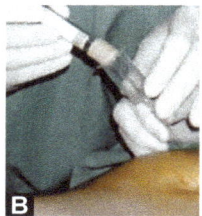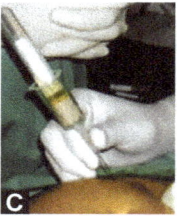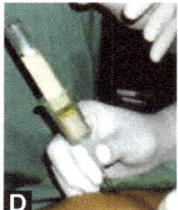

Figs. 8.2A to D: Step-by-step amniocentesis procedure.

Using an aseptic technique, a 20 or 22 gauge needle is inserted into the amniotic fluid under continuous ultrasound guidance. The tip and the shaft of the needle should be visible throughout the procedure. This reduces the incidence of bloodstained samples and should prevent damage to the fetus and/or the umbilical cord. Following removal of the inner stylet, and while doing so, the needle has to be static; care should taken not to push or pull the needle away from the free pocket of amniotic fluid localized. The syringe is carefully fixed to the hub of the needle and gently 18–20 mL of amniotic fluid is aspirated before the needle is removed under ultrasound guided from the uterus (Figs. 8.2A to D).

PRINCIPLE OF ULTRASOUND: IN PLANE APPROACH – NEEDLE BEAM ALIGNMENT

Needle beam alignment is very important and best achieved when needle is inserted in the same plane as ultrasound beam, this enables needle to be visible as a bright line, needle beam alignment is critical to visualize the entire shaft up to the tip of the needle. Needle should be advanced well guided and at an angle of 45° or less depending on the location of the target (Figs. 8.3 and 8.4).

For a successful invasive diagnostic technique, always scan just before you start the procedure. Identify the target, recognize the intervening structures. Procedure orientation is very important. This helps to decide on the type and length of the needle.

The transducer is held in the left hand of a right handed operator, the desired target is identified and the transducer is aligned in such a way that the target is in the center of the screen while the proposed site of entry in the maternal abdomen is visualized at the edge of the screen. Subsequently, the right index finger is placed

Amniocentesis

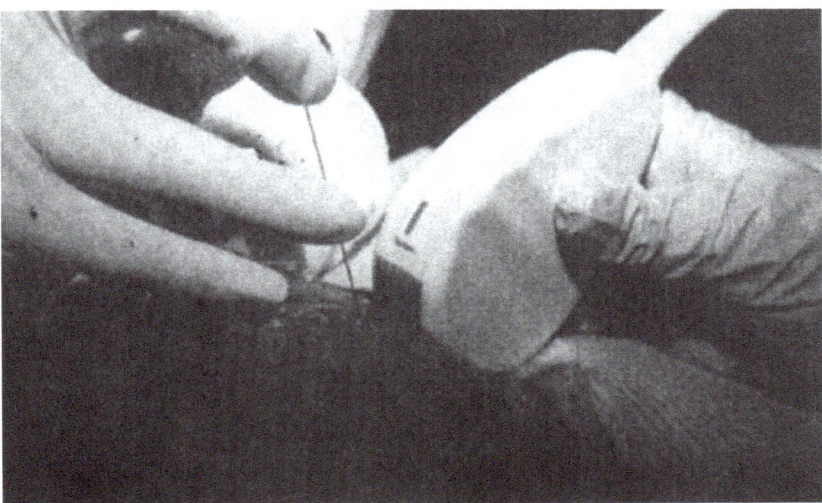

Fig. 8.3: Needle at 45°.

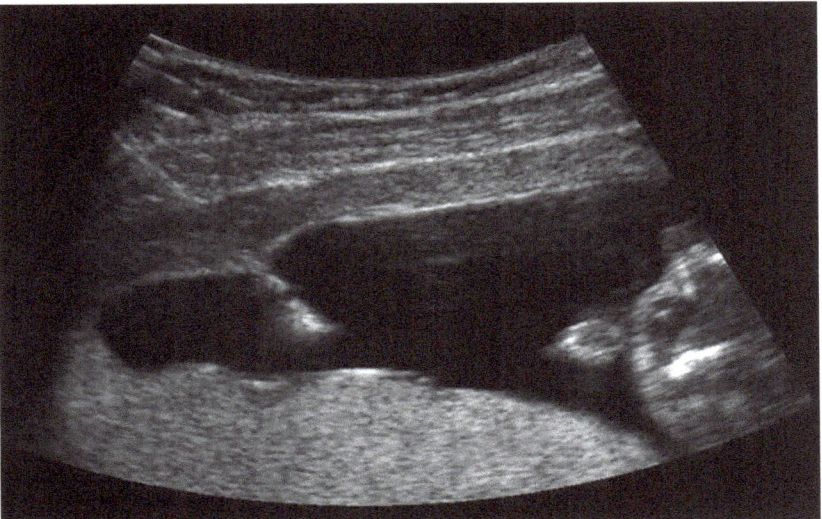

Fig. 8.4: Ultrasound needle beam alignment.

on the maternal abdomen, about 2–3 cm away from the edge of the transducer, and pressed firmly towards the uterus. Provided the finger and the transducer are within the same plane, the indentation caused is clearly visible, allowing the operator to simulate needle insertion. The needle or instrument is then introduced into the uterus, ensuring that the whole length is visualized continuously. This is best achieved when the needle is directed at 45° from the horizontal plane of the transducer.

During the procedure if the needle is lost, first stop advancing the needle. Locate needle by angulations of the probe, move probe and identify needle tip, finally move probe and needle together, under vision, back in line to the target. Thereafter fix the transducer and advance the needle as you see it, deeper you go, tracking and manipulating the needle will be painful, traumatic and difficult. Always remember to maintain the 45° angle while at the entry point and during advancing the needle.

All patients should have their blood group and rhesus factor checked before the amniocentesis. Those who are rhesus D-negative require taking 250 IU of anti-D immunoglobulin to prevent rhesus isoimmunization.

The amniotic fluid aspirated is bloody in approximately 1 to 2% of amniocenteses. The blood, which is almost always maternal in origin, does not adversely affect amniotic cell growth. Indeed, the performance of a transplacental amniocentesis may increase the risk for a bloody tap; this has not been shown to have an adverse effect on the safety or accuracy of the amniocentesis.

By contrast, brown or dark red or wine-colored amniotic fluid is associated with an increased likelihood of adverse pregnancy outcome. This color indicates earlier intraamniotic bleeding, with hemoglobin breakdown products accounting for the pigment. Pregnancy loss eventually occurs in about one-third of such cases. If the abnormally colored fluid is also characterized by an elevated AFP level, the risk for adverse perinatal outcome (fetal death, anencephaly, spontaneous abortion, or fetal abnormality) is usually further increased. Green amniotic fluid, presumably due to meconium staining, is apparently not associated with poor pregnancy outcome. By contrast, brown amniotic fluid has been associated with an increased risk of fetal aneuploidy.

Following amniocentesis, fetal heart motion should be documented by ultrasound visualization. The patient is observed briefly following the procedure and is instructed to report for any vaginal fluid loss or bleeding, uterine cramping, or fever. Reasonably normal activities may be resumed following the procedure; however, and coitus be avoided for a couple of days.

MULTIPLE GESTATIONS

In multiple gestations, amniocentesis can usually be performed on all fetuses, provided amniotic fluid volume is adequate. In experienced hands, amniocentesis is performed successfully in more than 95% of twin pregnancies with no increased risks over that of amniocentesis in singleton pregnancies.

Difficulties Encountered during Amniocentesis and How to Overcome

Amniocentesis appears to be a very simple procedure, and most of the time is performed quite smoothly. One should know that Amniocentesis may become eventful and is not without risks.

Amniocentesis can become difficult, or may encounter significant problems during the procedure.

Factors Predictive of a Difficult Amniocentesis Procedure

When there are uterine fibroids, more so on the anterior uterine wall, or in front of the desired point for entry of the needle. Presence of a fibroid offer resistance to the smooth passage of the needle also may result in bleeding from the fibroid and such injury may stimulate release of prostaglandins and therefore pain and contractions and increase risk of miscarriage following amniocentesis. Also the patient is uncomfortable and not cooperative during the procedure. Also increases time taken for the procedure.

In pregnancy where there are low levels of amniotic fluid, it may be difficult to get a reasonably good pocket of amniotic fluid to tap and will risk the fetal parts getting pierced. Also desired quantity of fluid will be difficult. In such situation you may have to locate the maximum pocket of fluid wherever possible, more so between the neck and thorax of the fetus or between the two femur bones or between the presenting part and the internal OS of the cervix. All these sites are not without risks to tap the amniotic fluid.

You may find the entire spread of the placenta on the anterior wall of the uterus, as already discussed, one may perform the procedure of amniocentesis by transplacental approach, while doing so, precaution should be taken to pierce and enter from the thinnest portion of placenta, avoiding the umbilical cord and the cord insertion at the placenta, for an uneventful experience.

Maternal obesity should not be underestimated, one may encounter difficulties in many ways. Firstly ultrasound evaluation may be difficult to evaluate fetal well-being and localization of a good pocket of amniotic fluid; ultrasound may not be able to visualize the entire needle, the shaft and the tip; lastly length of the needle may fall short and may not reach the desired pocket of amniotic fluid. In such situation it is very important to select the entry point, that is closest to the target and to measure the distances from the point of entry to the midpoint of a good pocket of amniotic fluid. This enables to decide the needle length to be used. If the length of the needle is not right, the maneuverability of the needle and reaching the desired pocket to get adequate amount of fluid is next to impossible.

There may be history of spotting or bleeding in current pregnancy, these situations are not to be taken lightly. One has to evaluate and re-evaluate to find the cause for such occurrences. One may require postponing the procedure if there is active spotting and treat the pregnancy. If one encounters any such events or injury resulting into bleeding raises the alpha fetoprotein. Also the possibility of getting abnormal prenatal diagnosis results, and the loss risks, are higher than those without such events.

Number of Needle Insertion

More than one needle insertion may be required in the following situations:
1. If the fetus moves and comes to lie close to or near to the site of needle entry, the needle may have to be pulled out and reinserted in a different spot to avoid injury to the fetal parts.
2. Difficulty getting the needle in, especially if the mother has a Braxton-Hicks contraction before or during the procedure. You may have to wait for such contraction to fade off and the needle has to be gently inserted.
3. Amniotic membrane 'tenting' occurs, where the membranes resist penetration by the needle and/or are pushed back but not penetrated by the needle. This may be more associated with fetuses with chromosomal abnormalities, more common in early amniocentesis procedures (Fig. 8.5).

Every needle insertion raises the risk, avoid multiple insertions whenever possible. Not more than two needle insertions in one

Amniocentesis

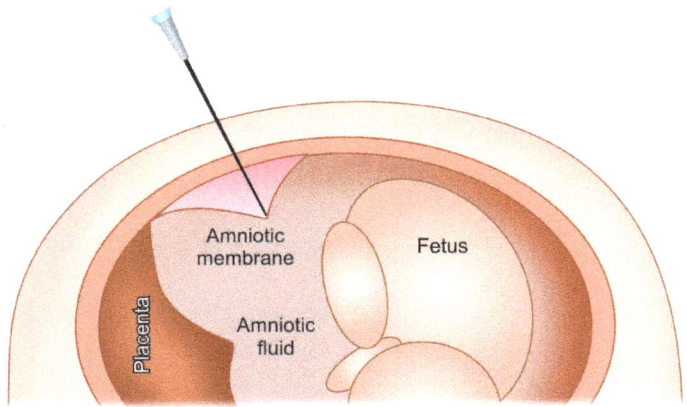

Fig. 8.5: Tenting of amniotic membrane.

amniocentesis session should be made. Amniocentesis should probably be abandoned that day and, if desired, tried again later to reduce the number of failed procedures and to reduce the fetal loss incidences.

BLOODY TAP

Bloody tap results from the needle insertion in the mother, from the skin, parities, uterine surface any extrauterine tissues and blood vessels. Also may occur when the placenta encountered, and finally may come from the fetus if injured. One should understand that problem amniocenteses have bloody taps associated with them more often, but a bloody tap alone does not necessarily mean there will be problems due to amniocentesis.

POSSIBLE PROBLEMS IN AMNIOCENTESIS

According to the March of Dimes, 1–2% of women experience cramping, spotting, bleeding, or leakage of amniotic fluid after an amniocentesis. Risk for miscarriage after a second trimester amniocentesis is 0.5–1%.

Reasons for Repeat Amniocentesis

1. Insufficient fluid or the fluid is contaminated by blood or maternal cells.

2. When laboratory is unable to culture enough cells from the amniotic fluid received and not able to do report Fluorescence in situ hybridization (FISH) and karyotyping.

Early Amniocentesis: Gestation of 14 Weeks or Less

With the advent of high-resolution ultrasound equipment, in an attempt to offer the option of early diagnosis, amniocentesis between 11 and 14 weeks of gestation has also been performed and evaluated.

Some programs not offering chorionic villous sampling (CVS) viewed early amniocentesis as an attractive alternative for those women who desired prenatal diagnosis before the time in pregnancy when traditional amniocentesis is performed (i.e. 15 or more weeks of gestation).

In other medical centers, early amniocentesis was explored to lessen the inconvenience of patient's having to be rescheduled if they came in for CVS and were determined to be beyond 12 weeks but under 15 weeks of gestation.

Loss rates were 7.6% for the early amniocentesis, post procedure amniotic fluid leakage occurred more frequently in the early amniocentesis group (3.5%) than in the midtrimester group (1.7%). Failed procedures, multiple needle insertions, and culture failures also occurred more frequently in the early amniocentesis.

Early amniocentesis has been reported to result in higher rates of birth defects such as Clubfoot (Talipes Equinovarus).

Early amnios have also been associated with a higher rate of fetal loss.

Largely early amnioceteses have been discredited as a viable prenatal testing technique therefore abandoned as an invasive prenatal diagnosis procedure.

AMNIOTIC FLUID SAMPLE COLLECTION AND TRANSPORT TO THE GENETIC LAB

Genetic Lab provided transport packing and transport system is the most suitable way of reaching the sample for prenatal diagnosis. Two to three conical test tubes with water seal screw caps placed in a slotted rack in a corrugated cardboard box. If 18 ml of amniotic fluid is required and collected, 6 ml of fluid should be filled in each of the three conical tubes. One should follow the checklist provided on the inner surface of the box before dispatching it to the lab. Place the referral letter with detailed history and stating the tests asked for. The duly signed informed consent and the PC-PNTD forms and the envelope of the specified charges for the tests required should be placed in the box (Figs. 8.6 and 8.7).

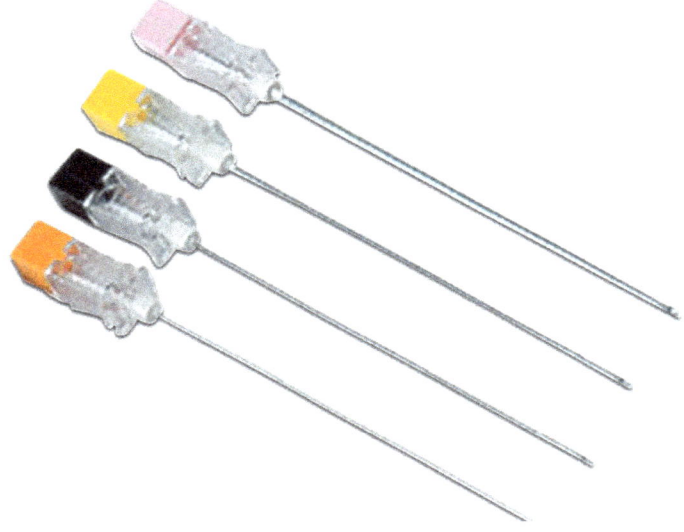

Fig. 8.6: Spinal needles.

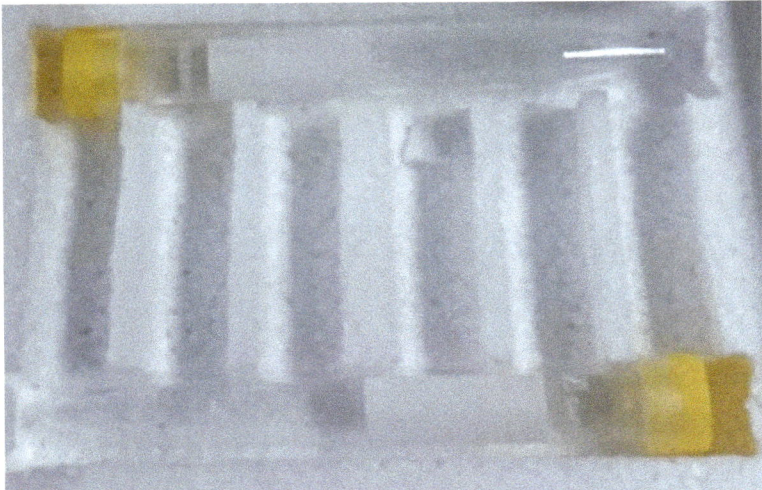

Fig. 8.7: Transport box.

CYTOGENETIC ANALYSIS

Amniocyte culture remains the gold standard for FISH and karyotype analysis.

Amniotic fluid samples are cultured over a period of 10–14 days. At this point the amniocytes are arrested during the metaphase stage of cell division, harvested, fixed on the slide and stained with dye. The visible chromosomes are then examined under the microscope. It may take up to 21 days to obtain a final report on the chromosome compliment. In addition to aneuploidy, examination of cultured amniocytes should also identify chromosome inversions, deletions and rearrangements.

To reduce the time delay in obtaining results for already anxious parents, newer techniques have been introduced. Fluorescence in situ hybridization (FISH) and quantitative fluorescence polymerase chain reaction (QFPCR) allow rapid evaluation of a small, selected number of chromosomes or chromosome markers but these techniques do not routinely identify more complex anomalies in the chromosome compliment.

While FISH and QFPCR offer a rapid diagnosis of trisomy 21, 18 and 13 or sex-chromosome abnormalities, other chromosome problems, such as rearrangements or deletions, will not be detected unless additional probes are specifically requested. For this reason, many laboratories still offer a full amniocyte culture report in addition to any rapid tests provided (Figs. 8.8 to 8.10).

SAFETY

Any procedure that involves passing a device into an organ, especially the pregnant uterus, entails risk; amniocentesis is no

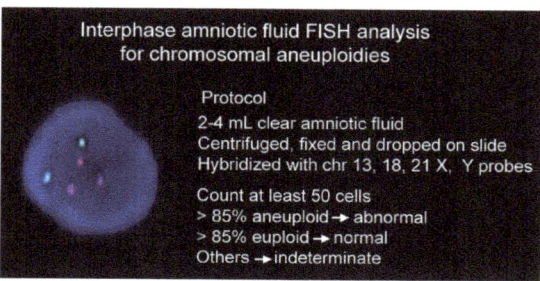

Fig. 8.8: FISH report.

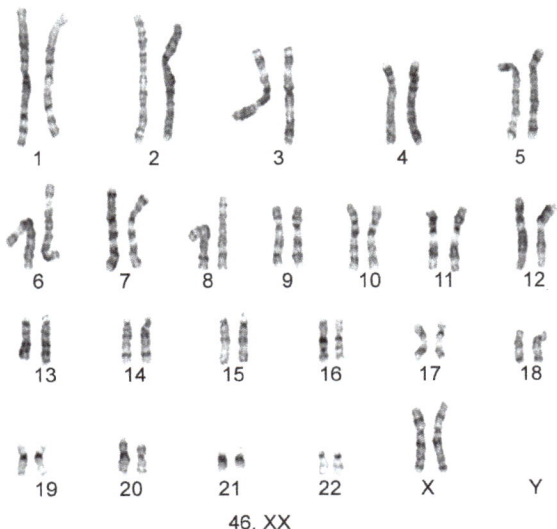

Fig. 8.9: Normal karyotype.

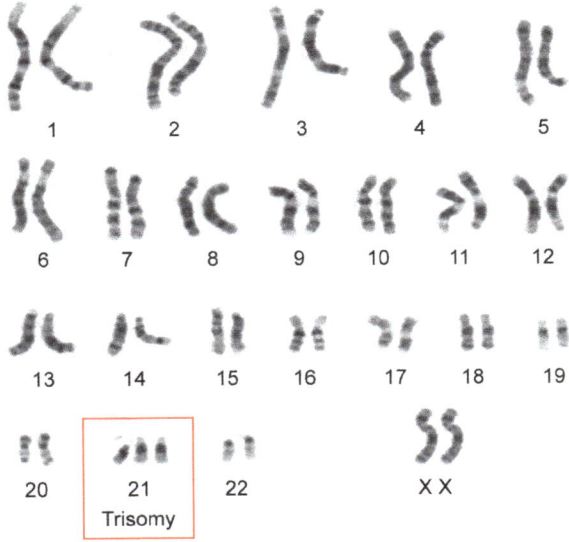

Fig. 8.10: Down syndrome karyotype.

exception. Indeed, amniocentesis carries potential danger to both mother and fetus. Maternal risks are quite low, with symptomatic amnionitis occurring only rarely. Minor maternal complications such as transient vaginal spotting and minimal amniotic fluid leakage occur in 1% or fewer cases, but these are almost always self-limited. Other very rare complications include intraabdominal organic injury or hemorrhage.

In conclusion, it is wise to continue to counsel that the risk of pregnancy loss secondary to amniocentesis is 0.5% over baseline, or perhaps slightly less at centers with experienced operators. Serious maternal complications and fetal injuries are stated to be 'remote' risks.

Chorionic Villous Sampling

INTRODUCTION

The technique of chorionic villous sampling (CVS) was first described as a means of first-trimester sex-chromosome determination in China. It was introduced into the West by a team at St Mary's Hospital in London and was subsequently developed during the late 1980s in Europe and America.

Kazy was the first to suggest ultrasound guidance to assist in safe biopsying the chorionic frondosum. Almost simultaneously, this approach was investigated and then modified by Humphrey Ward in London and refined by Bruno Brambatti in Milan.

Chorionic villous sampling is now a well-established procedure in prenatal diagnosis. The chorionic villi have same genetic constitution as that of the fetus and therefore reflects chromosomal, biochemical and DNA configuration of the fetus. CVS enables early, first trimester prenatal diagnosis and is a suitable alternative to amniocentesis. In addition to being safe, it also gives privacy of early diagnosis and making decision. CVS is reliable and offers widespread application. In experienced hands, CVS results in 99% sampling success.

This chapter discusses the standard techniques of CVS, both transabdominal and transcervical, as well as its safety and efficacy.

PROCEDURE RELATED ANATOMY

Gestational sac does not fill the entire uterine cavity. Chorionic member surrounds amniotic coelom. The villi over most of the chorion laeve are those that are degenerated and are forming the chorion laeve, while those villi remaining begin to embed into deciduas basalis, forming the chorionic frondosum, which will ultimately become the placenta (Figs. 9.1 and 9.2).

The individual chorionic villi float freely within the blood of the inter-villous space and are only loosely anchored to the underlying

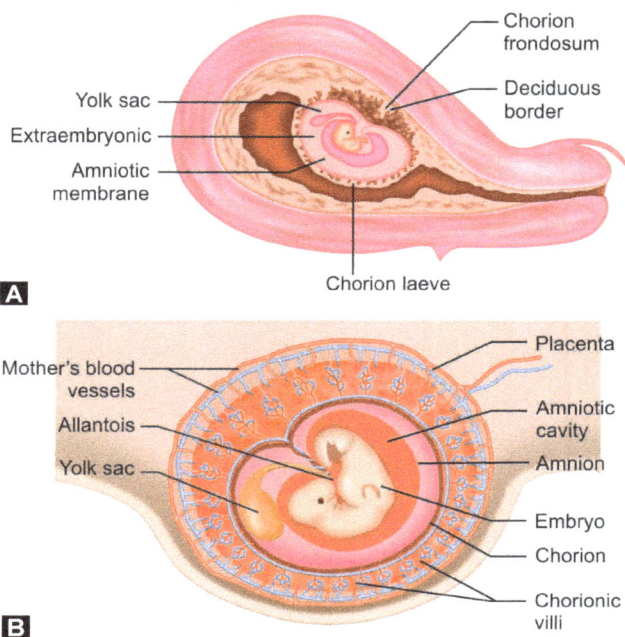

Figs. 9.1A and B: Procedure related anatomy.

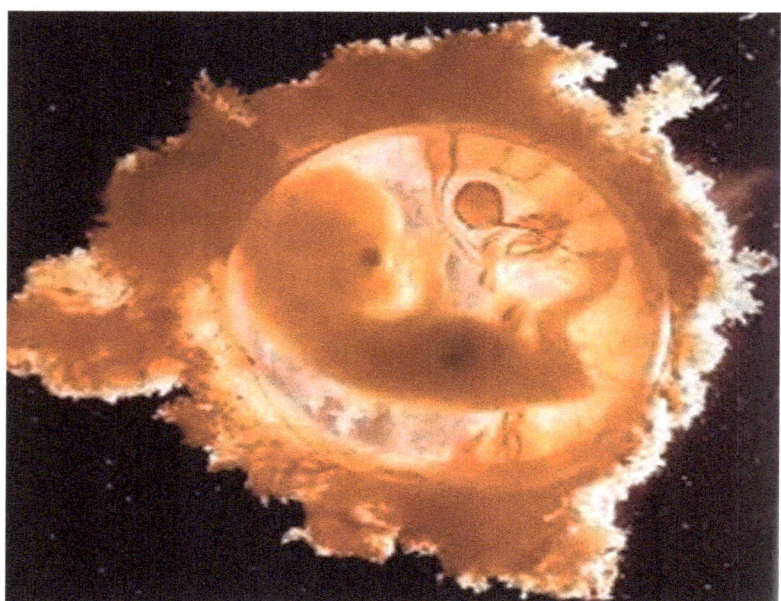

Fig. 9.2: Cord insertion and chorion frondosum.

decidua basalis. Chorionic frondosum villi are mitotically active, and, therefore, is the preferred biopsy site.

The surface of actively proliferating villi is punctuated by small buds consisting of an outer syncytial covering and a core of mitotically active cytotrophoblastic cells. Within the center of the villous is the mesenchymal core, through which capillaries carrying fetal blood cells course.

It is the cytotrophoblastic buds that provide the tissue for the direct preparation of karyotypes, while the embryologically distinct mesenchymal core serves as the source for tissue culture.

Preprocedure

All patients anticipating a CVS should rule out cervical infection, if present should be examined by smear and culture, and treated appropriately, more so those undergoing transcervical CVS. Also if erosion is present, the same should be treated and spotting and bleeding anticipated if held with a tenaculum.

Genetic counseling is mandatory prior to a CVS. The indication for referral is reviewed; alternative procedures are discussed for similar diagnosis. The patient should be informed of the potential risks and complications of the procedure as well as the limitations of genetic diagnosis.

In order to minimize patient anxiety, the practical aspects of the procedure should be explained in detail and the common complications that occur after the procedure, such as cramping, spotting and bleeding, should be outlined. Also testing versus no testing is discussed and informed written consent is taken before posting the patient for the procedure.

Clinical evaluation of the patient is of utmost important, which includes, a detailed Obstetric history, number gravidity, parity and abortions, mode of deliveries, number of surviving children. Family history of any affected child in either spouse families. One has to rule out any genital infection and treating the same prior to giving appointment for the procedure. Spotting of bleeding during current pregnancy make the procedure at high risk and should be asked for.

Prior to CVS, fetal viability and gestational age should be confirmed by ultrasound. The presence of twins as well as other pregnancy related pathology, such as subchorionic hematoma or a coexisting blighted ovum, could potentially affect the procedure and its interpretation and must be identified.

The procedure is best performed between 10 and 12 weeks. On the day of procedure, ultrasound is performed for confirming the earlier observation and orientation of the procedure, and uterocervical relation is reviewed. On ultrasound, frondosum appears as a hyperechoic homogeneous area and its location must be accurately determined prior to sampling. The umbilical cord insertion should be identified for confirmation.

The bladder should be sufficiently filled, and serves as an acoustic window, to allow adequate visualization of the entire sampling path; overfilling of the bladder should be avoided since it makes sampling more difficult. An overfilled bladder will push the uterus and thereby the cervix upwards high into the vagina, lengthen and stretches the cervix and make in-accessible to visualization and also limit uterine mobility making transcervical sampling difficult.

SAMPLING DEVICES

Transcervical CVS: This is performed with a polyethylene (Portex) catheter through which a metal malleable stylet is inserted. The outer sheath with an internal diameter of 0.89 mm. Portex cannula is expensive and disposable.

Transcervical CVS can be safely performed using stainless steel, malleable, economic, easy to autoclave, reusable cannula with an olive tip, that makes the cannula atraumatic and enable good imaging on ultrasonography, gauge 16, and length 20–22 cm. In addition, you require 10 cc, disposable syringe with transport medium (Figs. 9.3A to C).

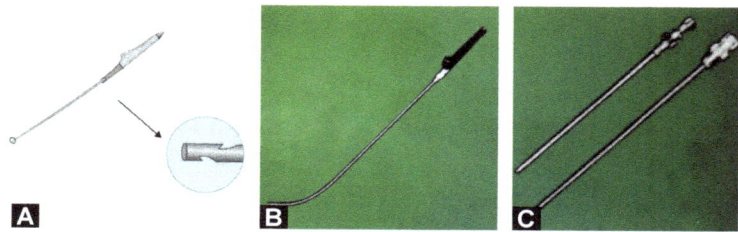

Figs. 9.3A to C: Devices used for transcervical chorionic sampling.

Chorionic Villous Sampling

Transabdominal CVS: Two techniques of sampling are presently used. In the single-needle approach, a 20 guage spinal needle is employed. In general, an 8–9 cm needle is sufficient for most samples but 12 or 15 cm needle should be available for very obese patients. Alternately, the double-needle technique uses an outer needle, a 18 gauge thin-wall needle. A smaller sampling needle, usually a 20 gauge, is then passed through the guide needle and used for the direct sampling. Once the needle is in place, a 10 cc syringe with transport medium is attached to the biopsy needle to achieve adequate negative suction. Some operators attach a hand grip or a low pressure mechanical suction and the collecting bottle to the biopsy needle (Figs. 9.4 and 9.5).

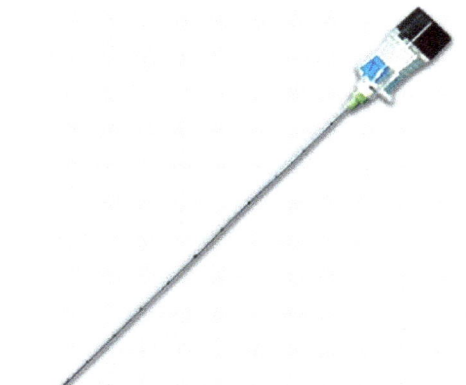

Fig. 9.4: Spinal needle.

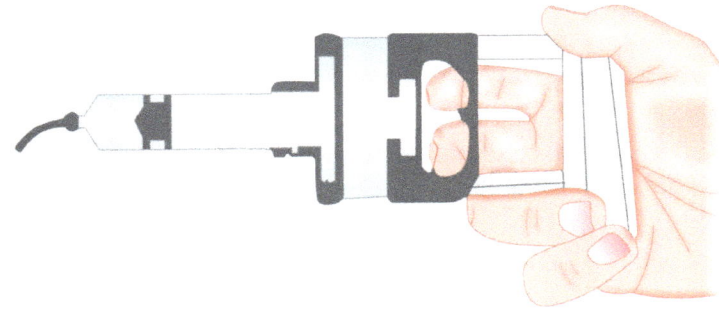

Fig. 9.5: Hand grip.

Common to both procedures are required transport culture bottle, Petri dish, lab suitable medium, vertical torch to identify good villi or dissecting microscope to study the villi and the coursing blood vessels through them.

Sampling Techniques

The selection of the route of approach, transcervical of transabdominal is really at the discretion of the operator and depends on the position of the uterus and the cervix and the uterocervical relation.

In fact, the route of approach largely depends on the site of location of the chorionic frondosum, the expertise of the operator, the facilities available at the center where the procedure is to be performed and finally the comfort and cooperation of the patient.

Presence of myomas on the anterior or lateral wall of the uterus would make a transabdominal approach painful, difficult and eventful. Again an acutely retroverted retroflexed uterus, also a cochleate uterus would require a long needle and would risk the depth of the needle insertion and encountering intervening organs and structures. Posterior location of chorion frondosum may become risky due to anteriorly presence of the fetus and the floating loops of the umbilical cord.

Both transcervical and transabdominal CVS are best performed using a two-person technique, with one individual performing the sampling and the other doing the ultrasound guidance. Communication and coordination between the sonologist and the operator is imperative and the best results are seen when number of team members are limited and fixed.

TRANSCERVICAL CHORIONIC VILLOUS SAMPLING

Transcervical route of procedure choice of, when obstetrician is the operator, being well-versed with the speculum examination, and the instrumentation. This route is counseled by them, is as easy as routine examination, as sounding of the cervix and uterine cavity, as placement of an intrauterine contraceptive device or as doing an intrauterine insemination, or even easier and safer, as it is under ultrasound guided (Figs. 9.6 and 9.7).

Chorionic Villous Sampling

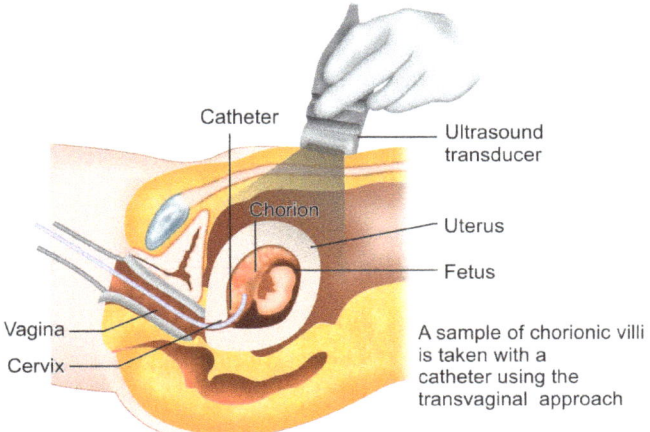

Fig. 9.6: Transcervical chorionic villous sampling.

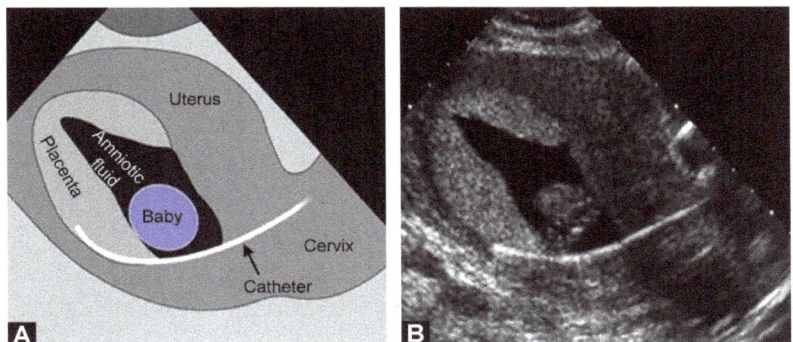

Figs. 9.7A and B: Diagrammatic representation and ultrasound appearance.

PRINCIPLES OF ULTRASOUND: THE ULTRASOUND BEAM

Understanding the ultrasound beam is of utmost importance. The thickness of the beam is limited to the thickness and stretch of the rubberized portion of the curved surface of the curvilinear probe forming a segment of visualizing window. This is comparable to visual restriction by the two eyelids to the ability of the eye to visualize. Only if the cannula is placed in this segment that it can be visualized at all time during the procedure by the guiding ultrasound transducer. Therefore, it is all about aligning ultrasound beam and cannula (Fig. 9.8).

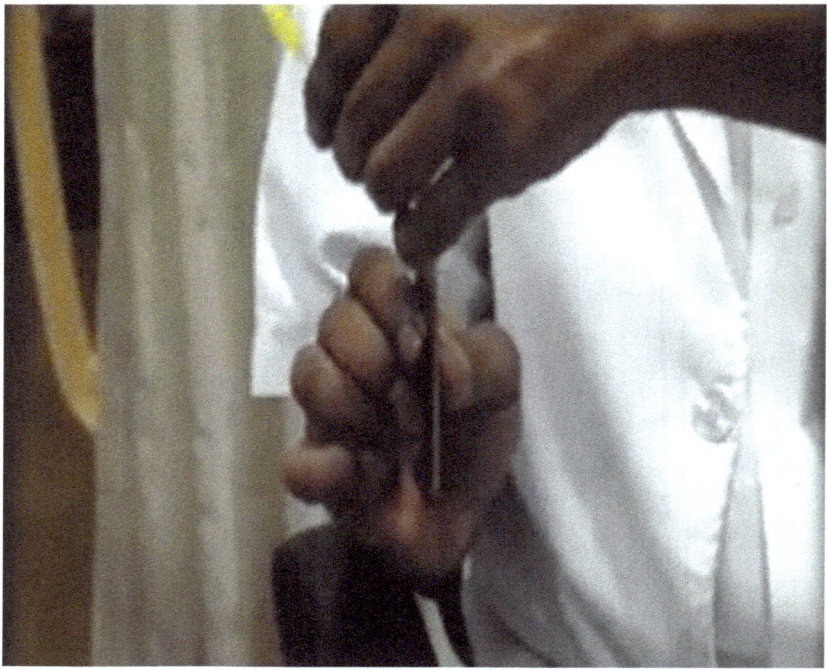

Fig. 9.8: Ultrasound beam.

The cannula has to be visualized throughout the procedure, at the entry, towards the target, reaching the target and at the time of exit. When these steps are followed, it truly defines and means that you have performed an ultrasound-guided procedure.

After ultrasound evaluation and orientation of the procedure, the patient is given lithotomy position, after aseptic precautions, a sterile vaginal speculum is inserted and the cervix directly cleaned with antiseptic.

Next tenaculum is placed on the anterior lip of cervix to stabilize the cervix and therefore the uterus. A gentle curve like, bend is given to the lower 2–5 cm of the catheter/cannula as per the ultrasound shown, the uterocervical relation and the mid-location of the chorionic frondosum to be reached. The cannula is then gently inserted through the cervix until the internal OS is reached. There is usually a slight loss of resistance at this point.

The further advancement is delayed until the sonographer is able to image the olive tip of the cannula. Once the cannula olive tip is through the internal OS, the tip must be pointed in the correct direction. An anterior position can be approached by pulling the speculum downwards, which will move the cannula tip upwards or by giving gentle traction to the tenaculun which will straighten the uterocervical angle and enable cannula to smoothly traverse anteriorly. A posterior approach is facilitated by rotating the cannula and its tip 180° downwards and then lifting the speculum. Once the tip is in place across the internal OS, the cannula is then gently advanced into the midst of chorionic frondosum.

Under direct visualization, the cannula should continue to be passed parallel and tangentially to the chorionic plate through the full length of the frondosum. Once in place, the stylet is removed, the 3–5 mL medium-filled, 10 mL syringe attached and approximately 3–5 mL of pressure applied. The cannula is moved 'to and fro' tangentially to the gestational sac, keeping the tip of the cannula in the midst of chorionic frondosum, because it is only the tip that will aspirate the villi, the villous tissue in the syringe barrel should be seen to be adequate and appears pinkish tissue, the cannula then removed in one gentle motion while suction is continuously applied. When the cannula is in the appropriate tissue plane in chorionic frondosum, there is no resistance to further advancement. The cannula should only be advanced using minimal pressure, if resistance is felt it indicates that the tip is either against the membrane or, more likely, within the deciduas.

The chorionic villi can be easily identified in the syringe by holding it up to a light. The villi are seen as free-floating, white tissue with fluffy, filiform branches. In contrast, decidual tissue has a more amorphous shape and lacks branches. The tissue so obtained is collected in the Petri dish containing the lab suitable medium. Now the Petri dish is placed either on the illuminated vertical torch or dissecting microscope and healthy villi are identified and confirmed.

If sufficient villi are not obtained on the first pass, a second attempt should be made. Pregnancy loss rate increases significantly when more than two insertions are required, and may be as high as 10% if three attempts are made. Therefore, third transcervical pass should be attempted when retrieval seems certain. Preferably, the cervical route should be abandoned and abdominal sampling should be considered.

DIFFICULTIES ENCOUNTERED AND HOW TO OVERCOME

Due to Cervical Factors

An undue long cervix would not allow the preformed, curved cannula to negotiate the internal OS and also decreases the cannula maneuverability.

A pin-point stenosed cervix, at external and internal OS may not allow the olive tip of the cannula to negotiate with ease, making the procedure painful and traumatic, resulting into noncooperation by the patient and spotting or bleeding of the cervix.

Presence of infected erosion on the cervix would carry risk of carrying infection to the pregnancy and undue bleeding of the erosion on touch (Figs. 9.9A to D).

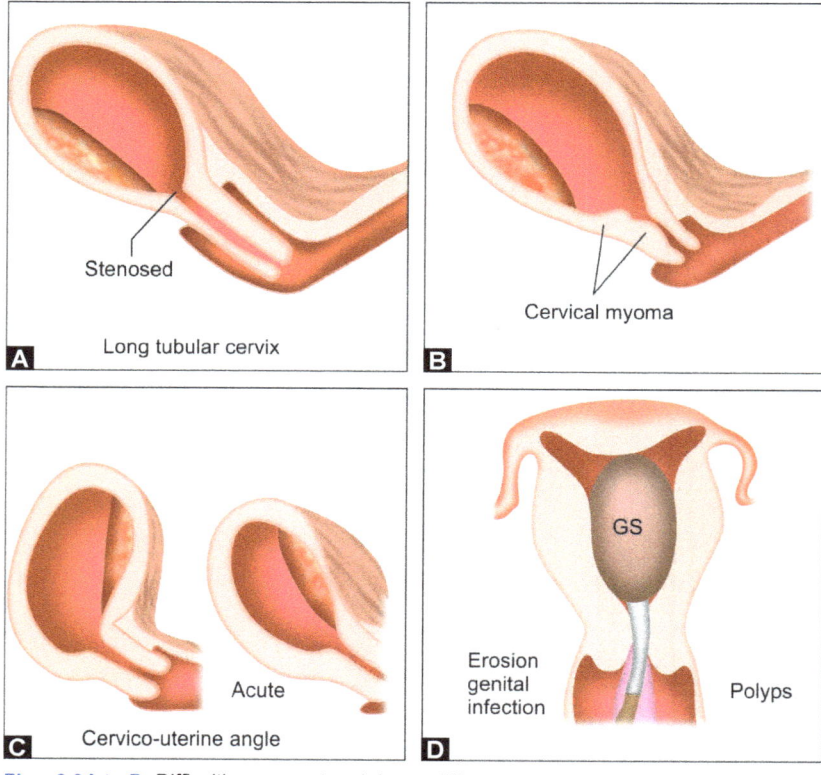

Figs. 9.9A to D: Difficulties encountered due to different types of cervical factors.

Due to Uterine Factors

Presence of uterine abnormalities, a retroverted fixed uterus would make maneuverability difficult in transcervical approach, a deviated fixed uterus would compromise ultrasound guidance.

An acutely anteverted anteflexed uterus as in a cochleate uterus, that is C-shaped uterus, passage of preformed curved cannula will be difficult (Figs. 9.10A to D).

Due to Chorion Frondosum

In early pregnancy, it is often seen the placement of chorionic frondosum at the internal OS, that is chorion low lying anterior or low lying posterior or chorion previa. It is wise to change the route of approach to transabdominal or postpone the transcervical procedure for 1–2 weeks awaiting migration of the low lying chorion.

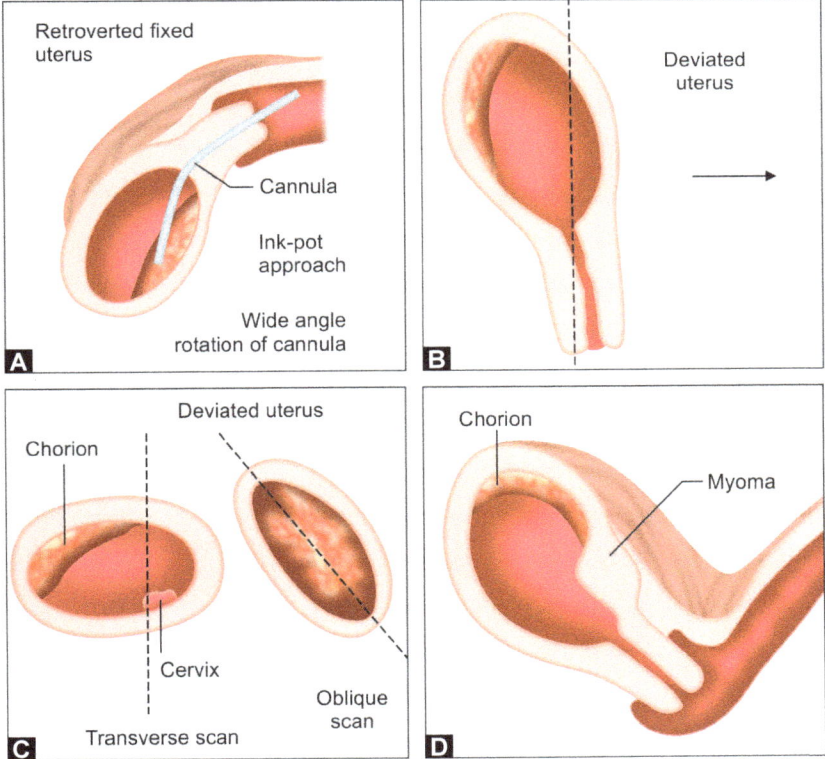

Figs. 9.10A to D: Difficulties encountered due to uterine factors.

Any intervention into low placed chorion would initiate bleeding, sometimes more the expected.

The thickness of chorion frondosumus is very important for its identification and obtaining adequate tissue sample. Lateral placement of chorionic frondosum make the ultrasound guided procedure more difficult in inexperienced hands.

Subchorionic hematoma, suggests separation of chorionic frondosum and make the procedure risky from fetal loss rate point of view. Such patient requires treatment, until the hematoma gets absorbed (Figs. 9.11A to D).

Due to Maternal Bladder

Adequately full bladder acts as an acoustic window to ultrasound beam. When the bladder is too full the cervix ascends higher and is located very high, making it difficult to localize and reach it.

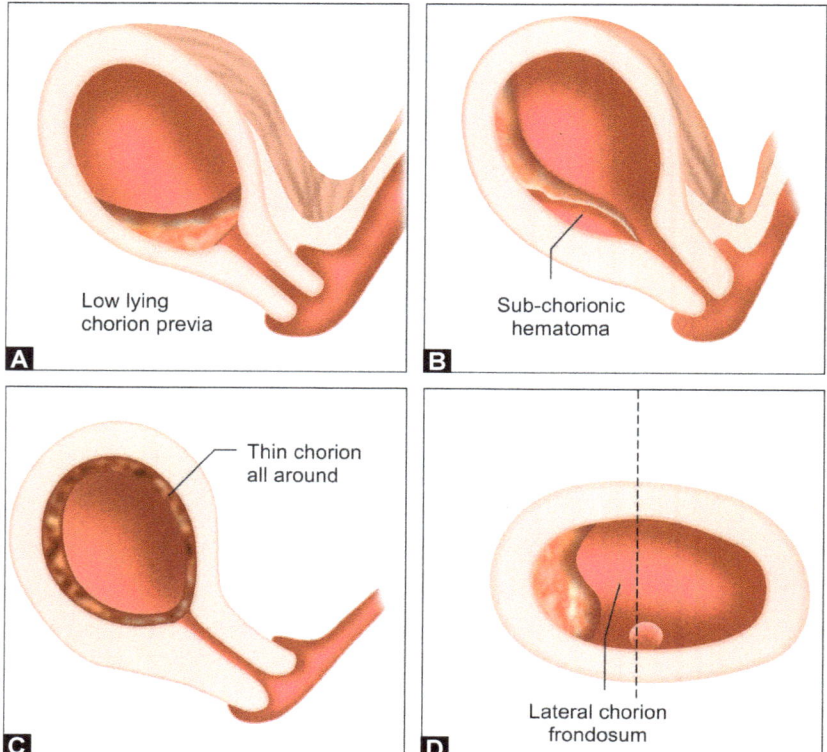

Figs. 9.11A to D: Difficulties encountered due to different kinds of chorionic frondosum.

Chorionic Villous Sampling

Most of the cannula length is utilized in reaching the cervix and therefore falls short in length in reaching the mid placed and fundally placed chorionic, frondosum. Also in such situation, maneuverability of the cannula is at stake.

Also a very full bladder fixes and restricts mobility of the uterus and thereby maneuverability and also may cause discomfort and pain due to ultrasound transducer pressure on the overt bladder.

Insufficient bladder results in poor imaging and guidance of the procedure. Also it exaggerates the cervicouterine angle, as if the uterus folding on the cervix, making difficult to confirm location of chorion frondosum whether on anterior or on the posterior wall of the uterus. Also makes cannula maneuverability impossible. The chorionic frondosum viewed as anterior wall is indeed on the posterior wall (Figs. 9.12A to D).

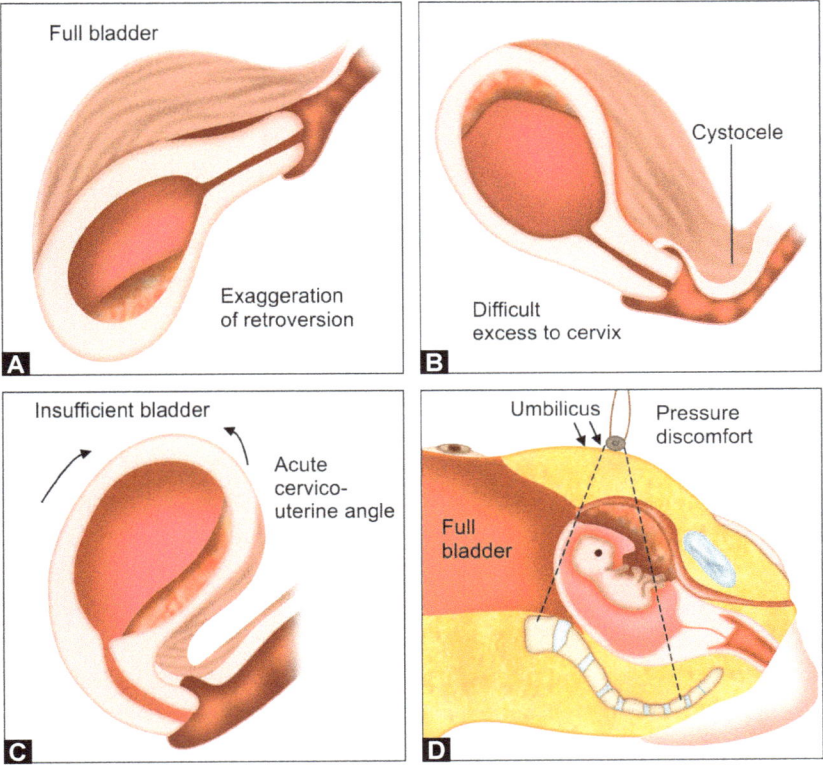

Figs. 9.12A to D: Difficulties encountered due to maternal bladder.

TRANSABDOMINAL CVS

The transabdominal route has become the technique of choice by the nonobstetrician operators, as it suits them both, the operator and the women. This route is counseled by them, has a lower rate of immediate complications, a lower risk of intrauterine infection and a shorter learning curve.

The abdomen is prepared with povidone iodine solution as for amniocentesis. The anticipated sampling path should be chosen such that the needle will pass parallel to the chorion frondosum and will avoid any intervening bowel and the gestational sac.

Transabdominal CVS could be performed using single needle technique or using double needle technique, these all perform equally well in experienced hands and the selection of technique used is therefore determined primarily by the operator's experience (Figs. 9.13 and 9.14).

Single Needle Technique

The chorion frondosum should be localized and seen to be accessible avoiding the gestational sac. A full bladder, which will usually push the uterus into an axial or slightly retroverted position, may facilitate access to an anterior placed chorion frondosum. Sampling a posterior chorion frondosum will generally be helped by asking the patient to empty her bladder, as the uterus adopts a more anteverted position.

If local anesthesia is used, this should be inserted under ultrasound guidance, through the abdominal wall to the level of the myometrium. Thereafter, taking a cue of the local anesthesia needle tract, an 18 gauge needle is progressively inserted through the layers of the abdominal wall and the myometrium until chorion frondosum is entered. Suction is applied via the aspirating syringe on the needle and attached syringe moved 'back and forth' resistance free, five to ten times within the chorion frondosum tissue. Following aspiration, seen as pinkish tissue and in adequate quantity, the needle and attached syringe are withdrawn under ultrasound guidance and the sample collected directly into culture medium on a vertical illuminated torch or dissecting microscope.

Chorionic Villous Sampling

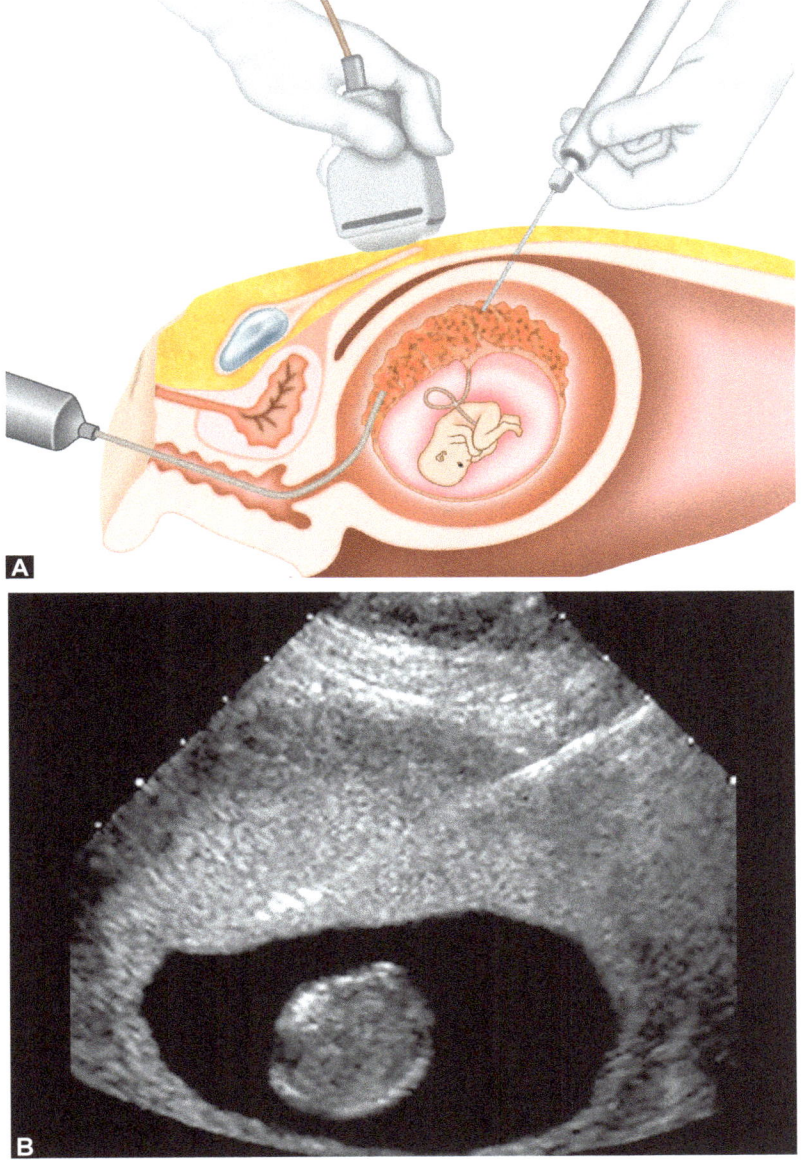

Figs. 9.13A and B: Diagrammatic and ultrasound images of transabdominal CVS.

The sample must be examined to ensure that a sufficient number of chorionic villi are present. If the sample is inadequate, the whole procedure must be repeated with reinsertion of the 18 gauge needle.

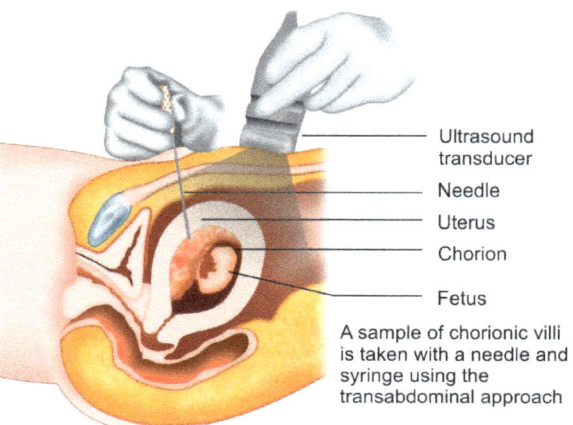

Fig. 9.14: Transabdominal CVS.

Double Needle Technique

An alternative approach is to use 'double needle' technique. The 18 gauge needle, once in the myometrium, is used as a 'guide' needle and a smaller 20 or 21 gauge needle inserted through the shaft. If repeat insertion is required, a double needle technique has an edge over the single needle technique.

COMPLICATIONS

As with amniocentesis, the greatest risk of CVS is pregnancy loss. The initial experience of CVS suggested the pregnancy loss rate to be at least 1-4%, greater than the loss rate associated with amniocentesis. As a result, there was little demand for the procedure.

Recent experience of CVS is more favorable. A systematic review of studies found the loss rate following transabdominal CVS (0.5%) to be almost identical to the loss rate following midtrimester amniocentesis (0.7%), and less the 1% following transcervical all invasive techniques.

Chorionic villoces sampling being more skillful, it is likely that the loss rate is much higher in less experienced hands.

In addition to fetal loss, an association with limb reduction defects, incomplete morphogenesis and disrupt normal embryogenesis is due to the vascular insult is of great concern. This was presumed to be due to placental microembolization occurring at the time of the procedure. A World Health Organization statement, following an analysis of 80,000 cases of CVS performed from 8 completed weeks onwards, failed to confirm these earlier findings but, in light of these risks, prenatal diagnosis by CVS is now usually performed beyond 10 weeks of gestation.

CONTRAINDICATIONS

Transabdominal CVS may be impossible to carry out if there are obstacles to the safe passage of the sampling needle, such as bowel attached to the abdominal wall or multiple fibroids. Transcervical CVS should not be carried out in the presence of vaginal or cervical infection. With either route, it is wise to postpone the investigation if there is active bleeding suggestive of a possible threatened miscarriage.

TIMING

The accepted gestational age for genetic CVS is between 10 and 12 weeks of gestation. The chorionic frondosum at this stage of pregnancy is easy to identify and of such thickness that safe sampling is usually possible. Although CVS can be carried out at later stages of pregnancy, second-trimester amniocentesis is generally preferred, because the technique is technically more straightforward, is deemed less uncomfortable for the woman and has a lower rate of mosaic results.

ASSESSMENT OF VILLI QUALITY

Chorionic villi from chorionic frondosum are pinkish tissue and appear distinctive frond like. They are branching type and have bud like projections on them. When seen under dissecting microscope, show blood vessels and capillaries coursing along them. These are live villi and readily grow when cultured (Figs. 9.15 and 9.16).

For cytogenetic analysis, quantity of villi required are 15–20 mg. Weighed when wet in medium.

Cytogenetic Analysis

The CVS sample is manually prepared, leaving clean chorionic villi for analysis. The sample is then either reported directly (a rapid result) or cultured before analysis.

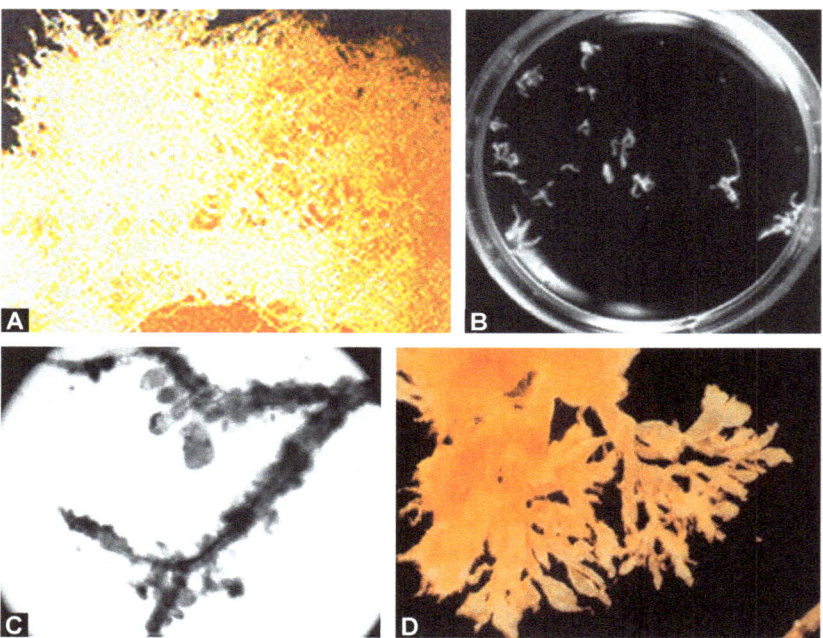

Figs. 9.15A to D: Vascular and mesenchymal structures of villi of chorionic frondosum.

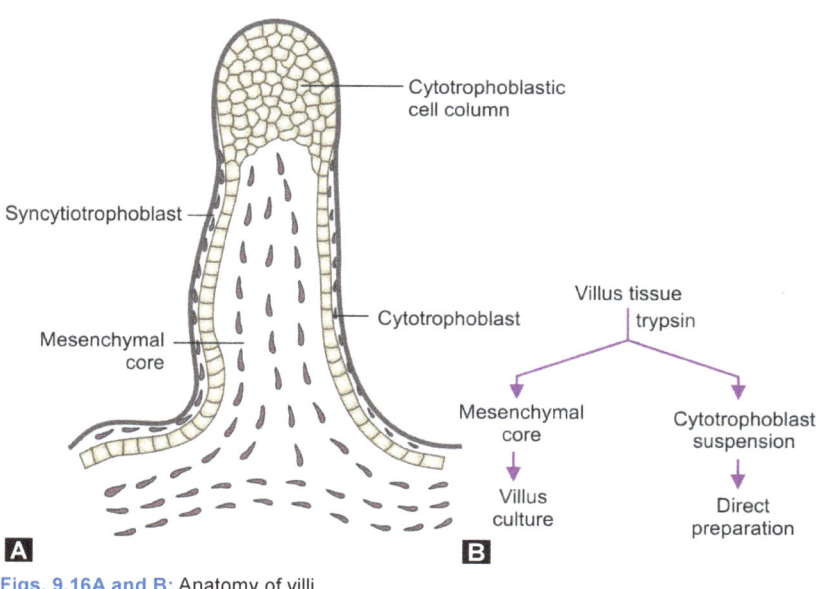

Figs. 9.16A and B: Anatomy of villi.

A rapid result FISH is obtained by examining cytotrophoblastic cells arrested in metaphase and a result usually available within 24–48 hours. A standard culture normally takes 10–15 days, after which time the mesenchymal cells are harvested and standard chromosome preparations obtained. Direct reports are associated with a small false-negative and false-positive risk and most laboratories therefore proceed with a full long-term culture to validate any preliminary or rapid reports.

Chorionic villous sampling diagnosis is only possible on the assumption that the chromosome complement of the fetus and chorionic tissue are identical. This is true for the vast majority of pregnancies but, occasionally, different cell lines are found in the fetus and chorionic tissue, a condition known as confined mosaicism. This condition occurs in 1–2% of all CVS samples and necessitates further testing in the pregnancy. True mosaicism, the presence of two or more cell lines within one fetus is extremely rare.

As with amniocentesis QFPCR and FISH are now used to speed up the diagnosis of aneuploidy in CVS specimens. Chorionic villi are also suitable for investigations other then cytogenetic analyses: the tissue is metabolically active and can thus be used in the diagnosis of many inherited metabolic diseases. The amount of DNA obtained from conventional sample, allows for many analyses using recombinant DNA technology. Such analyses are not usually possible with amniotic fluid cells.

CHAPTER

Cordocentesis

Cordocentesis as a method of fetal blood sampling was first carried out in the 1960s under fetoscopic guidance and carried a procedure-related fetal loss rate of over 5%. The first percutaneous umbilical cord sampling under ultrasound control was reported by Daffos et al.

In 1983 this development revolutionized the technique, allowing access to the fetal vascular compartment for both diagnostic and therapeutic means, with a procedure-related fetal loss rate of less than 2%.

Owing to the introduction of FISH and QFPCR, fetal blood sampling is rarely used to test for aneuploidy in current practice but it may be required to evaluate of fetal karyotype if a mosaic result is obtained or there are inconclusive results following CVS or amniocentesis.

Cord blood sampling still has a place in the investigation of fetal infection and the anemia that can follow infections such as parvovirus, congenital toxoplasmosis and rhesus isoimmunization.

TECHNIQUE

The umbilical vein is identified ultrasonically and, using a free-hand technique, a 20-gauge spinal needle is inserted under direct ultrasound control. The procedure is technically more difficult and the loss rate higher if the procedure is carried out before 20 weeks of gestation. The site of cord insertion at the placenta, where the cord is relatively fixed, is the most favored target for cordocentesis. Local anesthesia is not generally used (Figs. 10.1 and 10.2).

Using ultrasound principles, the needle is guided to the umbilical cord through the placenta, that is transplacental

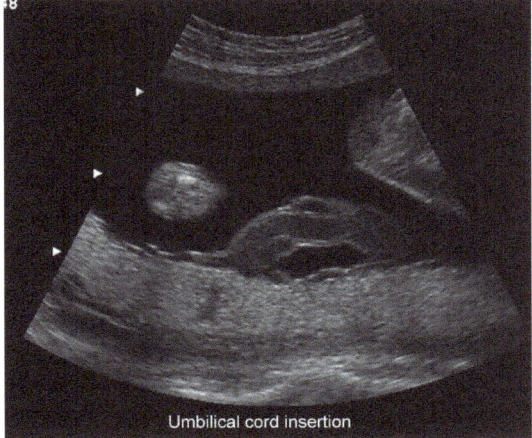

Fig. 10.1: Identification of umbilical vein by ultrasound.

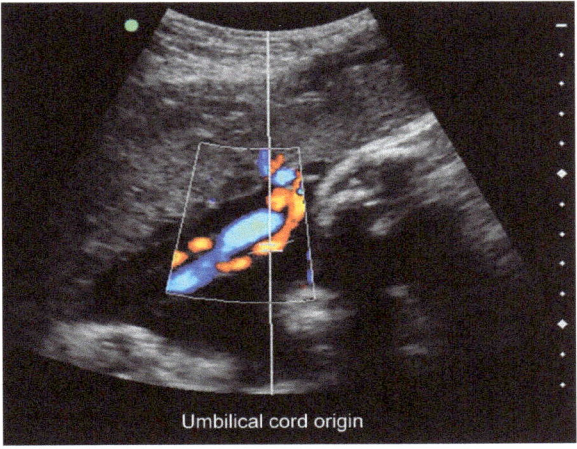

Fig. 10.2: Color Doppler confirmation of cord origin.

approach or through the amniotic cavity, that is transamniotic approach of the cord insertion in the amniotic cavity (Figs. 10.3 to 10.6).

COMPLICATIONS

The major complications of cordocentesis are fetal bradycardia, bleeding at the puncture site or occasionally asystole. The world experience of cordocentesis is much smaller than for other invasive techniques such as CVS or amniocentesis.

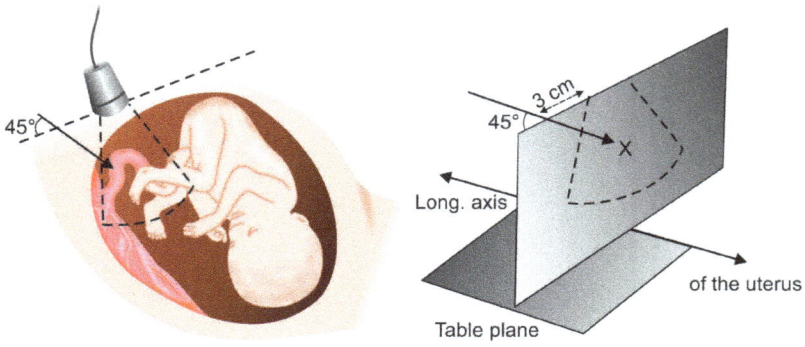

Fig. 10.3: Ultrasound principle cordocentesis.

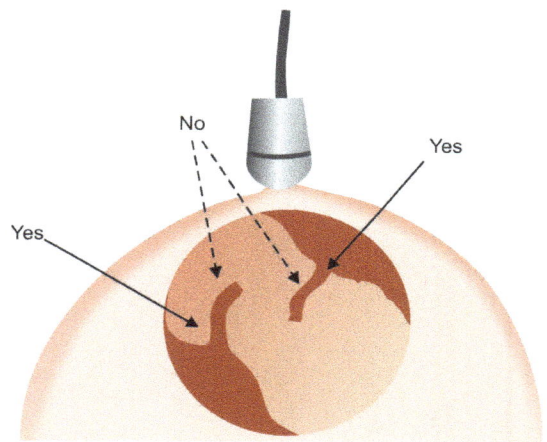

Fig. 10.4: Transplacental and transamniotic approach.

WHICH PROCEDURE AT WHICH GESTATION?

Transabdominal or transcervical CVS is the diagnostic technique of choice in pregnancies of less than 12 weeks of gestation. In experienced hands, there is minimal risk of pregnancy loss and failed or mosaic cultures are rare. It remains a technically demanding procedure requiring extensive operator experience to achieve competency. In pregnancies of greater than 14 weeks of gestation, mid-trimester amniocentesis and/or placental biopsy is the preferred procedure. It is technically less complex, has a very low risk of pregnancy loss in experienced hands and has very few

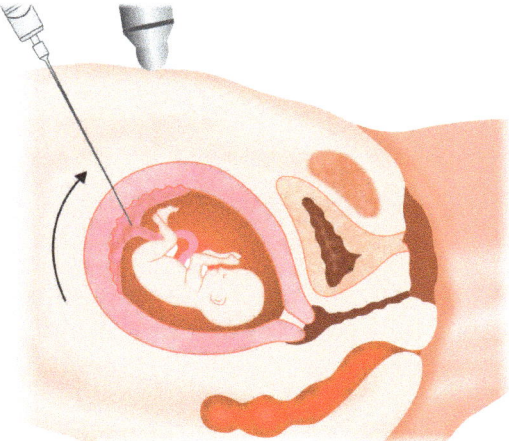

Fig. 10.5: Transplacental approach of the cord insertion.

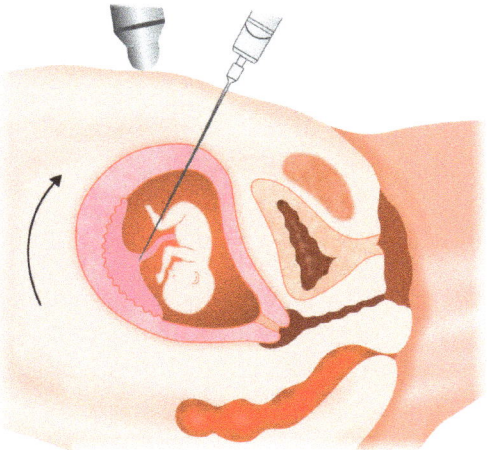

Fig. 10.6: Transamniotic approach of cord insertion.

additional risks. Owing to the technical limitations and improvements in the speed of cytogenetic analysis, cordocentesis is now reserved for specific or difficult diagnostic dilemmas.

Embryoscopy

Embryoscopy is a relatively new and investigational technique that permits direct visualization of the fetus as early as the first trimester. Initially, a rigid fiberoptic endoscope was passed transcervically into the extracoelomic cavity, permitting inspection of fetal anatomic structures; fetal blood sampling was also feasible by this method. However, improvements and advancements in fiberoptic technology have led to the performance of thin-gauge transabdominal and transcervical embryoscopy, allowing visualization as early as 4 weeks after conception (Figs. 11.1 and 11.2).

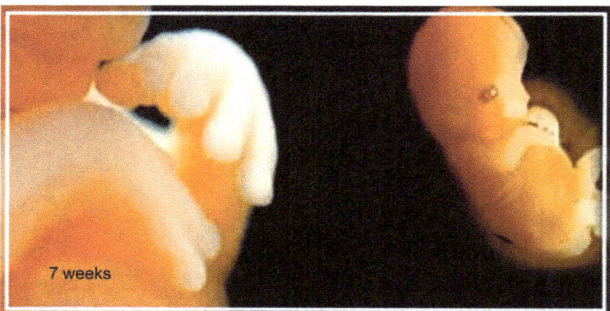

Fig. 11.1: Early embryoscopy at 7 weeks.

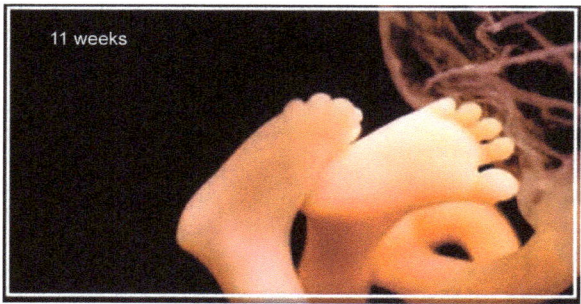

Fig. 11.2: Embryoscopy at 11 weeks.

Initial procedures were performed only on women who had elected pregnancy termination; however, embryoscopy has since been performed on continuing pregnancies. Ville and colleagues reported a procedure-related loss rate of 12% when the procedure was performed in the first trimester.

Further studies of the safety, accuracy, and applications of this new modality will be needed before embryoscopy is used as a routine prenatal diagnostic tool. However, the ability to access the embryonic circulation may have important application for therapeutic interventions such as drug, gene, and cell therapy.

Multiple Pregnancy and Prenatal Diagnosis

Diagnostic testing in women with a multiple pregnancy is a complex clinical scenario that raises major ethical dilemmas for parents; in particular, the options for pregnancy management in that event only one fetus to be affected.

Multiple pregnancy testing require specific counseling, with special mention of difficulties encountered, requiring separate route of approach depending on location of the target site. The possibilities of diagnostic errors should be informed. The patient should be informed about vanishing of one of the twin.

Gestational age and fetal biometry is very important. If the fetal ages are discordant there is a small risk of vanishing of the smaller fetus. Such fetuses are identified and their placement noted diagrammatically in view of requirement of selective termination if found to be abnormal.

The procedures for multiple pregnancies should be performed using separate sets of devices. Goes without saying the samples collected should be packed and labeled carefully.

Careful ultrasound guided procedures should be done, taking care not visiting the same sac and fetus. One should limit aspiration of fluid as in case of amniocentesis in the midst of amniotic pocket. In chorionic villous sampling, one has to limit the movements of the tip of the cannula or needle within the chorionic frondosum, to ensure sample from the desired gestation sac.

The results are matched with the labeled gestation sac and counseled with the patient. If selective termination is requested for one has to be very careful in identifying the abnormal fetus.

AMNIOCENTESIS

The relative location of each gestation sac and placenta must be carefully documented. Although sampling both gestation sacs using a single-needle insertion has been described, there are theoretical concerns about sample mixing, failure to adequately puncture the inter-twin membrane and therefore failure to truly sample both sacs and potential damage to the inter-twin membrane.

Many clinicians therefore use a double-needle insertion using the technique previously described for CVS or sample each gestation sac using a separate needle insertion point for each sac.

It is critical that the samples obtained are precisely labeled, to ensure that the result can be accurately linked to the correct gestation sac, thus avoiding a fetal error if selective termination is indicated.

There is wide variation in the reported post-procedure loss rate in multiple pregnancies, ranging from 0 to 3% greater than the background rate.

CHORIONIC VILLOUS SAMPLING

CVS in a multiple pregnancy is a technically demanding procedure. In a monochorionic twin pregnancy, some parents will request that only one sample is obtained but they must be aware that ultrasound-determined chorionicity may not be 100% accurate for all other multiple pregnancies, the chorionic frondosum positions must be clearly mapped and documented, to ensure that each chorionic mass is sampled. In addition, the operator should note whether the bladder is full or empty, as this can significantly alter how each gestation sac and chorion appear to be positioned. Separate needles should be used to prevent cross contamination of the samples (Figs. 12.1A and B and 12.2).

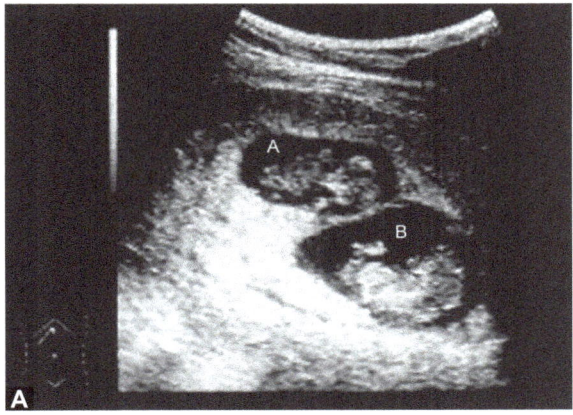

Fig. 12.1A

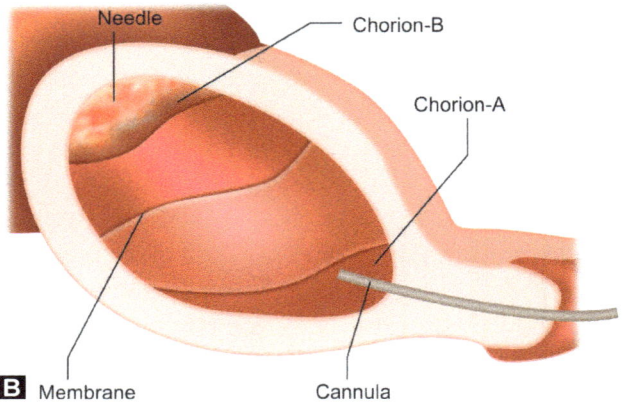

Figs. 12.1A and B: Ultrasonography evaluation of TWIN gestation.

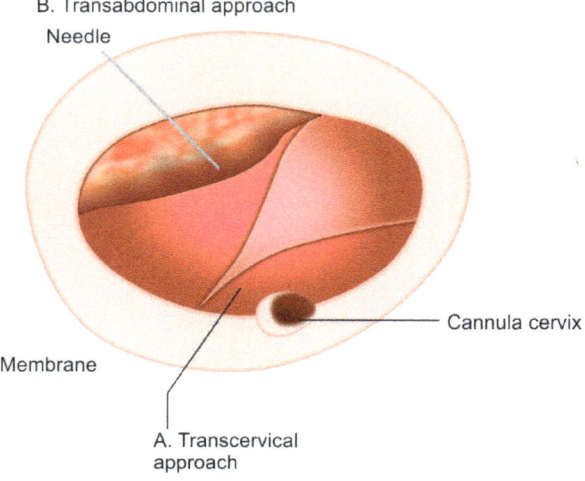

Fig. 12.2: Diagrammatic representation of TWIN gestation.

The samples must be labeled in such a way that each result can be matched to the appropriate fetus.

As for amniocentesis, there are limited data available on the loss rate following CVS in multiple pregnancies but it would appear to be no different to the background loss rate for twin pregnancies. There is an increased risk of sampling error and mosaicism during CVS in multiple pregnancies. With experienced operators, the risk of sample error is greatly reduced.

CHAPTER 13

Summary and Suggested Reading

SUMMARY

Invasive prenatal testing remains a mainstay of obstetric practice in the United States. When provided within a framework of nondirective genetic counseling and supportive follow-up, invasive testing can provide critical information to women and couples concerning pregnancy outcomes. However, effective genetic counseling and follow-up as well as extensive clinician training and procedure evaluation is needed to provide best prenatal diagnosis to women at increased risk for detectable fetal abnormalities. It is hoped that further advances will facilitate access to the fetus and help develop safer invasive procedures.

The development of diagnostic ultrasound has opened the field of invasive ultrasound-guided procedures with numerable applications. The free-hand, two-operator, end-on technique is preferred. Local anesthetic is used in complex procedures but not in routine procedures. Prophylactic antibiotics are used only in high-risk situations. Developing skills and technique with simulators will be helpful to gain confidence. The most important aspect of all invasive procedures is experience and teamwork between operator and sonologist.

- In the years to come, the demand for a high quality fetal medicine and therapy will steadily increase, due to the growth of the three factors:
  (1) the continuous improvement in diagnostic and therapeutic capabilities, (2) the increasing perception of the fetus as a person, resulting from better and more accurate imaging techniques, and (3) increasing public awareness and demands for advanced fetal medicine and therapy solutions, in the context of the global information society.
- The development of imaging techniques and of molecular medicine will allow diagnoses and treatments today unimagined.

- The clinical use of noninvasive prenatal testing to screen high-risk patients for fetal aneuploidy is becoming increasingly common. Initial studies have demonstrated high sensitivity and specificity, and there is hope that these tests will result in a reduction of invasive diagnostic procedures as well as their associated risks.
- The clinical use of noninvasive prenatal testing to screen high-risk patients for fetal aneuploidy is becoming increasingly common. Initial studies have demonstrated high sensitivity and specificity, and there is hope that these tests will result in a reduction of invasive diagnostic procedures as well as their associated risks.
- Invasive diagnostic procedures are there to be in late maternal age, with positive family and medical history, when biochemical and or noninvasive prenatal screening (NIPS) tests indicate high risk.
- Invasive procedure chorionic villous sampling, amniocentesis and cordocentesis for routine karyotyping, FISH and for chromosome microarray studies.

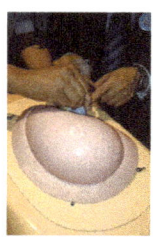

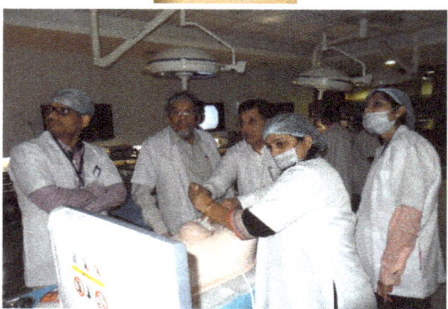

I believe

'See one, Do one, Teach one'

This will not only help perfect one's own technique but also will make utilization of 'invasive techniques for prenatal diagnostic technique' safe and practiced by many more.

SUGGESTED READING

The **Pre-natal Diagnostic Techniques (Regulation and Prevention of Misuse) Act**, PCPN-DT Act 1994 **Lee P Shulman, MD,** *Professor Gynecology and Molecular Genetics; Director, Division of Reproductive Genetics, Department of Obstetrics and Gynecology, University of Illinois at Chicago, Chicago, Illinois*

Joe Leigh Simpson, MD, *Ernst W. Bertner Chairman and Professor, Department of Obstetrics and Gynecology, Baylor College of Medicine, Houston, Texas*

Sherman Elias, MD, *Henry and Emma Meyer Chair in Obstetrics and Gynecology, Professor, Obstetrics and Gynecology, Professor, Molecular and Human Genetics, Director, Division of Reproductive Medicine, Baylor College of Medicine, Houston, Texas*

Prenatal Diagnosis: **past, present, and future,** Authors, Malcolm A. Ferguson-Smith, Diana W. Bianchi, First published: **22 June 2010**

Fetal Medicine for the MRCOG and Beyond, *Alan Cameron, Janet Brennand, Lena Crichton, Janice Gibson, editor Jenny Higham*

Ultrasound in Obstetrics & Gynecology, *by Narendra Malhotra, PK Shah, Prashant Acharya, Sonal Panchal, Jaideep Malhotra*

ISUOG Practice Guidelines: invasive procedures for prenatal diagnosis T. Ghi, A. Sotiriadis, P. Calda, F. Da Silva Costa, N. Raine-Fenning, Z. Alfirevic, G. McGillivray

Prenatal Diagnostic Techniques, *Prashant Acharya, S Suresh, Deepika Deka, Pratima Radha Krishna, Anita Kaul, Narendra Malhotra, Jaideep Malhotra, Ashok Khurana, P K Shah, Mandakini Pradhan, Geeta Kolar, Suseela Vavilala, Chander Lulla, Hema Diwakar, Gokul Das*

Principles and Practice of Fetal Medicine, *Raju R Sahetya, Hema Purandarey, Jaideep Malhotra, Ankesh R Sahetya, Divya A Sahetya*

Interventional Ultrasound in Obstetrics, Gynaecology and Breast *Ultrasound-Guided Techniques in Fetal Medicine, Kypros H Nicolaides, Yves Ville*

Interventional Ultrasound in Obstetrics, Gynaecology and Breast, *Chorionic Villous sampling, Ronald J Wapner*

Interventional Ultrasound in Obstetrics, Gynaecology and Breast, *Amniocentesis, Luis F Goncalves, Roberto Romero, Hernan Munoz, Ricardo Gomero, Maurizio Galasso, David Sherer, Jose Cohen, Fabio Ghezzi*

Prenatal Diagnosis in Obstetric Practice, *Whittle and Connor*

Chorionic Villus Sampling, *Liu, Symonds and Golbus*

Limb abnormalities and chorionic villus sampling. *Lancet 337: 1423, 1991 Jackson LG, Wapner RJ, Brambai B:*

Techniques and safety of genetic amniocentesis and chorionic villus sampling. *Elias S, Simpson JL In Sabbagha RE (ed): Diagnostic Ultrasound Applied to Obstetrics and Gynecology, p 113. 3rd ed. Philadelphia, JB Lippincott, 1994*

Embryoscopy: New developments in prenatal diagnosis, *Reece EA: Curr Opin Obstet Gynecol 4: 447, 1992*

A short history of Amniocentesis, Fetoscopy and Chorionic Villus Sampling, *Dr. Joseph Woo.*

INDEX

Note: Page numbers followed by *f* refer to figure.

A

Alpha-fetoprotein (AFP) 11
American Congress of Obstetricians and Gynaecologists (ACOG) 5
Amniocentesis 5, 35, 72
Amniotic fluid 36
Analysis of amniotic fluid 11
Anatomy of villi 64*f*
Anencephaly 38
Aneuploidy 3
Anomaly scan 5
Aseptic technique 36
Assessment of villi quality 63

B

Biopsy forceps 13
Bloodstained samples 36
Bloody Tap 41
Brown amniotic fluid 38

C

Cardiac abnormalities 2
Chorionic frondosum 34
chorionic tissue 8
Chorionic villous Sampling 12,47
   preprocedure 49
   procedure related anatomy 47
   sampling devices 50
   sampling techniques 52
Transabdominal CVS 51
   transcervical CVS 50
Chromosomes for diagnosis 3*f*

Congenital diaphragmatic hernia 2
Contingent test 4
Cordocentesis 8, 14, 66
   complications 67
   procedure 68
   technique 66
Counseling prior to invasive prenatal diagnostic procedure 16
Curvilinear probe 27
Cystic hygroma 2
Cytogenetic analysis 44, 63
Cytotrophoblastic cells 8

D

Diagnostic techniques 3
Diagnostic testing 2
Double-needle insertion 73
Down syndrome 4
Down syndrome karyotype 45*f*
Duodenal atresia 2

E

Early amniocentesis 42
Embryofetoscopy procedure 15
Embryoscopy 15, 70
Ethical issues 18

F

Fetal abnormality 38
Fetal biometry 72
Fetal blood sampling 14
Fetal cell 8

Fetoscopy 14
First trimester ultrasound 4
FISH analysis 44*f*
Fluorescence in situ hybridization (FISH) 44
Free-hand techniques 22
  'end-on' approach 23
  'parallel' or 'side-on' approach 22
  perpendicular offset approach 22

G

Genetic amniocentesis and diagnosis 11
Genetic counseling 16
Gestational age 72
Gestational sac 47

H

Holoprosencephaly (HPE) 2
Human chorionic gonadotropin (hCG) 6

I

Inborn errors of metabolism 11
In plane technique 28
International society for prenatal diagnosis (ISPD) 4
Inter-twin membrane 73
Invasive diagnostic procedures 7
Invasive prenatal diagnostic technique 3
Invasive prenatal testing 1
Invasive procedures 7

L

Legal issues 19

M

Malleable cannula 34
Malpractice lawsuits 19
Meckel-gruber syndrome 15

Mesenchymal cells 8
Multiple gestations 39
Multiple pregnancy 72

N

National society of genetic counsellors (NSGC) 5
Needle beam alignment 29, 36
Needle-guide adapters 12
Neural tube defects 11
Neural tube screening 4
Noninvasive prenatal screening (NIPS) 5
Normal karyotype 45*f*
Nuchal translucency 4
Number of needle insertion 40

O

Optimal prenatal testing protocol 4
Out of plane technique 28

P

Paradigm shift in prenatal diagnosis 6
Percutaneous umbilical blood sampling (PUBS) 14
Phospholipid 11
Pre-conception and prenatal diagnostic techniques (PCPNDT) Act 3
Principle of ultrasound 36, 53
Procedural prerequisites 33
  clinical evaluation 33
  pregnancy evaluation 33
  ultrasound evaluation 33
Procedure orientation 32
Prostaglandins 39

Q

Quad test 4
Quantitative fluorescence polymerase chain reaction (QFPCR) 44

Index

R

Repeat amniocentesis 41
Retroflexed retroverted uterus 34
Rigid fiberoptic endoscope 70
Risk of miscarriage 39

S

Specific chromosome abnormality 2
Sphingomyelin 11
Sphingomyelin ratio 11
Spinal needles 43*f*
Spontaneous abortion 38

T

Technical aspects 20
Touch technique amniocentesis 21*f*
Transabdominal CVS 60
  complications 62
  contraindications of CVS 63
  double needle technique 62
  single needle technique 60
Transcervical cannula 34
Transcervical chorionic villous sampling 52
Transport box 43*f*
Tricks and tips for a successful procedure 31
Trophoblast villi 13

U

Ultrasound beam 25, 36
Ultrasound principles in invasive prenatal diagnostic procedure 23
Umbilical vein 15

X

X-linked conditions 11

www.ingramcontent.com/pod-product-compliance
Ingram Content Group UK Ltd.
Pitfield, Milton Keynes, MK11 3LW, UK
UKHW051958200326
4879IPUK00007B/108